# Stepping into Palliative Care 1

## Relationships and responses

## Second Edition

Edited by

## Jo Cooper
*Macmillan Clinical Nurse Specialist in Palliative Care*

Foreword by
## Reverend Professor Stephen Wright
*Faculty of Health and Social Care*
*St Martin's College, Carlisle*
*Chairman, The Sacred Space Foundation*

Radcliffe Publishing
Oxford • Seattle

**Radcliffe Publishing Ltd**
18 Marcham Road
Abingdon
Oxon OX14 1AA
United Kingdom

www.radcliffe-oxford.com
Electronic catalogue and worldwide online ordering facility.

───────────────────────────────

© 2006 Jo Cooper

Jo Cooper has asserted her right under the Copyright, Designs and Patents Act 1998 to be identified as author of this work.

New research and clinical experience can result in changes in treatment and drug therapy. Readers of this book should therefore check the most recent product information on any drug they may prescribe to ensure they are complying with the manufacturer's recommendations concerning dosage, the method and duration of administration, and contraindications. Neither the publisher nor the author accepts liability for any injury or damage arising from this publication.

All rights reserved. No part of this publication may be reproduced, stored in a retrieval system or transmitted, in any form or by any means, electronic, mechanical, photocopying, recording or otherwise, without the prior permission of the copyright owner.

British Library Cataloguing in Publication Data

A catalogue record for this book is available from the British Library.

ISBN-10: 1 85775 793 9
ISBN-13: 978 1 85775 793 4

Typeset by Advance Typesetting Ltd, Oxford
Printed and bound by TJ International Ltd, Padstow, Cornwall

# Contents

# Foreword

I grew my hair long, wandered around Europe and did all those things you were supposed to do in the 1960s. But as they drew to a close and that decade slipped into the 70s, it was time to get serious; paternal pressure pushing me further into conformity and the search for a steady job. And so I found myself in Matron's office at my local hospital being given the third degree about becoming a nurse. She did not hide her scepticism about me making it – as a man and grammar school educated to boot, I was clearly not made of the right stuff. The next intake of students was four months away. Meanwhile, 'I'm sending you to geriatrics and the chronic sick ward,' she commanded. 'If you can survive that you can survive anything.'

Thus my introduction to nursing was a ward full of people, mostly but not all elderly, in various stages of decay and dissolution, where the only way out was on the mortuary trolley. Where not-always-so-tender loving care was about all that was on offer.

Times have changed.

Palliative care and its twin sister hospice care are well established on the map. The speciality continues to expand and deepen its knowledge and practices into territory undreamed of even a few decades ago. My first ward experience left me with deep appreciation of the sheer gutsy hard work of most of the staff in the face of appalling resources, dreadful conditions and levels of despair and suffering that would make lesser mortals shrivel away. It also left me feeling, 'There has to be a better way than this.'

This book (which needs to be read with its sibling book *Stepping into Palliative Care 2: care and practice*) offers the better way, rooted in the burgeoning fields of research and scholarly enquiry that now form the foundations of effective palliative care. It explores dimensions which many aspects of care in my early years of nursing universally ignored – the caring relationships, the emotional responses of patients and carers, and the search for meaning, support and healing in the maelstrom of the human experience of palliative care. As caring professions involved in palliative care began to deepen and expand their knowledge and practices several decades ago, there was much emphasis, quite rightly so, on what worked best for patients. Yet there was less emphasis on what the staff needed in this speciality, not just practical knowledge and skills but also the therapeutic and relational awareness of their roles, their needs as individuals and in teams and as part of wider organisations. If we know what good quality palliative care is, and we do, then what is needed to support it? What sort of organisation works best to meet patients' needs? What personal and ethical dilemmas need to be solved? What makes therapeutic relationships effective for patients and nurturing for the carers?

These and other related questions are explored in this book, giving emphasis not just on what the patient experiences, but also what the professional carer goes through as well. These themes are woven into each chapter as the best of palliative care for both patients and carers is illuminated. While there is extensive use of up-to-date research, this is not just a text to read and inform, but also to stretch and engage. We also learn by participating so, dear reader, you are invited by every contributor to step beyond the comfort zone of merely absorbing and participate in the self-assessment exercises in each chapter. Our creativity in palliative care is enhanced when our own thinking is stretched beyond its usual boundaries through reflection and enquiry. And reflective, enquiring, creative, compassionate, expert carers are going to be needed even more for this speciality, for it too is seeing its boundaries stretched and its practices challenged and endlessly reforged. That chronic sick ward, in a peculiar way, was a harbinger of modern palliative care, for it was filled not just with terminally ill cancer patients, but with people in end-stage 'senility' (as it was called then) or multiple sclerosis, the profoundly disabled stroke patient or the post-trauma brain damaged. Then it was the ward of hopeless cases; now they and more like them are the landscape into which palliative care is expanding.

And it is not only the diagnostic reach that is being stretched, but also the possibilities of care for each individual. For, as this text embraces, our awareness of the needs, for example, of ethnicity and sexuality has to become part of our everyday practice if care is to be truly holistic and integrated. The infinite possibility of caring needs professional carers who are gifted with an immense range of knowledge and skills, who have personal insights to know their own strengths, limitations and needs and of those with whom they work in the caring milieu. This book informs, involves and invites all those who work in palliative care to be expert, compassionate, insightful human beings ready, able and willing to be with those in need.

Stephen Wright
*August 2006*

Rev. Professor Stephen G Wright FRCN MBE
Faculty of Health and Social Care, St Martin's College, Carlisle
Chairman, The Sacred Space Foundation
Editor, *Spirituality and Health International*
steve@sacredspace.org.uk
www.sacredspace.org.uk

# Setting the scene

The first edition of *Stepping into Palliative Care* was primarily intended for those new to the field of palliative care. The second edition is aimed at a broader readership, crossing all role boundaries and differing levels of expertise. Within *Stepping into Palliative Care 1: relationships and responses* and *Stepping into Palliative Care 2: care and practice* there are many new chapters not only addressing the practical, technical and fundamental care issues but looking deeper and wider into *how* being a person with cancer, and the family, feels. Issues of existentialism, the human experience of *being,* and the nature of therapeutic relating, have been comprehensively embraced. *Stepping into Palliative Care 1 and 2* can be applied to practice by the novice and experienced practitioner, and aim to present illustrations of best theory and practice.

As palliative care travels its own unique and distinctive voyage, the significance of attending to the spiritual, social, emotional and psychological needs of the patient and family are paramount in the provision of care. This second edition looks at not only the need for empirical knowledge, but also the aesthetic knowledge, and art of caring. It aims to capture the essence of what it *means* to be *alongside* suffering: care that goes beyond words, capturing souls, spirit and compassion.

It is essential to remember the *true* meaning of palliative care in a time where we are politically conscious of the need to demonstrate clinical effectiveness and to determine outcomes of care. Two opposing paradigms, on one continuum: *both* can be met and intertwined.

In order to meet the requirements of the individual who is exposed to palliative care, the professional needs education and training targeted at the *how to* element of professional practice and patient management. For the professional who is in daily or occasional contact with the patient, family and significant others affected by cancer, it is an integral part of his or her professional daily life. For the professional to be able to identify problems and monitor treatment, interventions and support services, it is essential there is a clear pathway of perception of the active role that each one of us plays, and participates in – be that before, during and/or after palliative care has been accessed.

In *Stepping into Palliative Care 1 and 2*, each chapter builds on the last to offer an overview of the needs relating to the individual who encounters palliative care. Where applicable, a chapter makes full and effective use of *at-a-glance* features including boxes, tables, figures, self-assessment, reflection and case scenarios. The *'To learn more'* sections point the reader in the direction of further knowledge and information. At the end of the book there is a *'Useful contacts'* section that can provide more information, advice and guidance for the professional, patient, family and significant others.

This edition can be used as a starting point to further education and training. It attempts to provide some sensitive answers, discuss some issues surrounding palliative care, and direct the reader towards further development.

*If you lose hope, somehow you lose the vitality that keeps life moving, you lose that courage to be, that quality that helps you go on in spite of it all. And so today I still have a dream.* (*The Trumpet of Conscience,* Martin Luther King, Jr)

Jo Cooper
*August 2006*

# Cautionary note

Throughout this book, reference is made to drugs and dosage. The authors and editor have made every effort to check the accuracy of this information and to ensure that information is up-to-date. However, it should be noted that drugs, dosage and indications can change as current research and developments provide new supporting evidence. It is essential that the prescribing individual check the drug, dosage and indications, at the time of the proposed prescribing, with current recommendations. Moreover, the individual administering the medication should check the evidence available at that time. The pharmacist is a valuable resource for all aspects of drug administration and prescribing information. The editor would recommend cross-referencing from the latest edition of Twycross R, Wilcock A, Charlesworth S *et al. Palliative Care Formulary* (Radcliffe Publishing).

# List of contributors

## Editor

Jo Cooper BSc (Hons) (Palliative Nursing), Dip Oncology, RGN, Specialist Practitioner – adult nursing (palliative care)
Macmillan Clinical Nurse Specialist in Palliative Care
Winkleigh, Devon

## Contributors

**Phil Barker**
Visiting Professor, Trinity College Dublin

**Poppy Buchanan-Barker**
Director, Clan Unity International
Newport on Tay, Fife

**Anne Bury** MA, BA, PGCE, RGN, RSCN
Head of Education
North Devon Hospice
Barnstaple, North Devon

**Sheila Cassidy** BM, BCh, MA (Oxon), DSc (Hon), DLit (Hon), DMed (Hon), UKCP
Psycho-Oncologist
Plymouth

**David B Cooper**
**Jo Cooper**
Winkleigh, Devon

**Professor Robin Davidson** MSc (Clin Psych), DPhil, ABPS
Consultant Clinical Psychologist
The Northern Ireland Cancer Centre
Hon Lecturer, Queens University, Belfast
The Gerard Lynch Centre
Belfast, Northern Ireland

**John E Ellershaw** MA, FRCP
Director, Marie Curie Palliative Care Institute, Liverpool
Clinical Director, Directorate of Palliative Care, Royal Liverpool University Hospitals
Professor of Palliative Medicine, University of Liverpool

**John Fletcher-Cullum** BSc (Hons), RGN
Clinical Nurse Manager
North Devon Hospice
Barnstaple, Devon

**Jon Hibberd** BSc (Hons), Dip HE, RN
Clinical Nurse Specialist in Palliative Care
North Devon Hospice
Barnstaple, North Devon

**Angela Jones** RGN, RM, RHV, BSc (Hons)
Team Leader/Clinical Nurse Specialist
North Devon Hospice
Barnstaple, North Devon

**Carol Kirby** MEd, BPhil (Hons), DN (London), RNT, RGN, RMN
Senior Lecturer
Faculty of Life and Health Sciences
University of Ulster at Magee
Northern Ireland

**Jonathan Koffman** MSc, BA (Hons)
Lecturer in Palliative Care
Guy's, King's and St Thomas' Schools of Medicine
Department of Palliative Care and Policy
King's College London

**Helen Meehan** RGN, RM, BSc (Hons) (Community Health Nursing)
National Lead Nurse, GSF
Lead Nurse Palliative Care, Solihull PCT

**Vicky Robinson** MSc, RGN, DN
Nurse Consultant
St Christopher's Hospice
Sydenham, London

**Mary Ryan** BA, MB, BCh, MRCGP, FRCP
Consultant in Palliative Medicine
North Devon Hospice
Barnstaple, North Devon

**Oliver Slevin** RGN, RMN, RNT Dip, BA, MA, PhD
Lecturer/Director: Doctor of Nursing Science Programme
School of Nursing
University of Ulster at Jordanstown
Northern Ireland

**Keri Thomas** MB, BS, DRCOG, MRCGP, MSc (Palliative Medicine)
National Clinical Lead Palliative Care (Generalist)
NHS End of Life Care Programme
Clinical Director Community Palliative Care, Birmingham
GP with Specialist Interest Palliative Care, Eastern Birmingham PCT
Honorary Clinical Senior Lecturer, Birmingham University

# Acknowledgements

To each author for their rigorous hard work, dedication, passion and commitment in producing quality text for *Stepping into Palliative Care 1 and 2* despite continuous heavy workloads. For completing chapters willingly, sharing knowledge, expertise, personal knowledge and experience and adding to the richness of this second edition – thank you.

Thank you to Gillian Nineham for having faith in me, and to Lisa Abbott, Jamie Etherington, Paula Peebles and the team at Radcliffe Publishing.

To the chapter reviewers for their expertise and constructive comments: Susanna Hill, Louise Whitehead, Sue Lloyd, Claire Taylor, Sheena McCullough and Philip D Cooper – thank you.

To my immediate team colleagues who have provided a source of strength, inspiration, vision, wisdom and encouragement – thank you.

To David, my advisor, administrator, greatest critic and my best friend, without whom what follows would never have been.

Any errors and omissions are the sole responsibility of the editor.

Jo Cooper
*August 2006*

# Dedication

Where my journey into palliative care began ...
... to the nurses and medical staff of the bedded unit, St Nicholas Hospice, Bury St Edmunds, West Suffolk.
... and to where the journey continues ...
... to the nurses and medical staff of the bedded unit, North Devon Hospice, Barnstaple, Devon ...
... special people, who touch our lives in a certain way, and having known them, we will never be the same. **Thank you.**

To our third generation – our hope for the future ...

*We should not let our fears hold us back from pursuing our hopes.*

(John F Kennedy)

**Jo Cooper**
*August 2006*

# Chapter 1

# Learning to learn in palliative care

*Anne Bury*

> *It is the self aware palliative care nurse who, with a blend of expertise, intuition, creativity and compassion, can make the experience as bearable as possible for the patient and his or her family.*[1]

---

**Pre-reading exercise 1.1**
**Time: 30 minutes**

- What do you think is necessary to provide good palliative care?

Think of a time when you were either a patient or carer and remember a health professional that you felt really understood and connected with your needs.

- What was it about this person; what knowledge, skills and qualities did s/he have?
- How do you think s/he learnt them?

Now, think back to the first patient you looked after who died.

- What sticks out in your mind?
- What support was offered to the patient, family and yourself?
- Did you feel prepared?
- What education and training had you received?
- What knowledge do you think you needed?

---

## How do you learn in palliative care?

Palliative care embodies the art and heart of healthcare. Learning palliative care and to feel comfortable with dying is a complex and lifelong endeavour. Palliative care is more than just learning how to fix a problem. As people come to the end of their lives, patients, families and colleagues need us to be alongside them, one human being to another. It requires us to learn the art of connecting, as whole person to whole person, soul to soul. This can present us with a challenge given the increasing emphasis on measurement, targets, outcomes, the medicalisation[2] of palliative care and the continued existence of ritualised and task-based practices in day-to-day care.

As you read this chapter, imagine that you are going on a journey. You will be wearing special rose-coloured lenses to help challenge and question yourself and your understanding of palliative care, education, training and learning. Reflect on what you already know and consider important. Explore your:

- feelings
- values

- attitudes
- experiences.

Consider:

- how you learn
- from whom you learn
- what stops you learning
- what you need to unlearn.

## Why is learning palliative care important?

For many years, education about death and palliative care has been neglected in nursing and medical education and training. What there is has been largely ineffective.[3–6] Evidence highlights the need for us to learn:

- pain and symptom management[7,8]
- physical care
- communication issues
- how to handle difficult questions and conversations with dying people[9]
- how to handle emotions[10,11]
- how to deal with ethical and moral dilemmas[12]
- how to acknowledge our own mortality.[13]

The need for palliative care is increasing with the rise in the numbers of older people and those with cancer and non-malignant illness. Thankfully, this need has been recognised in recent government documents. The National Service Frameworks (NSFs) and the NICE (National Institute for Health and Clinical Excellence) guidance on supportive and palliative care[14] recommends that those providing generalist and specialist palliative care receive the necessary knowledge and skills to provide it.

## Key areas of knowledge in palliative care

The practice of palliative care is an art and science. The two are intertwined, and both are essential. However, over recent years scientific knowledge and technical aspects, such as symptom management and outcome measurement, have received greater legitimacy and emphasis.[15]

Seminal research[16] identified several aspects of palliative care work that illustrate the breadth of knowledge we need, most of which are linked to the art of care (*see* Figure 1.1).

Both the *three kinds of knowing* (*see* Box 1.1)[17] and *four patterns of knowing* (Box 1.2)[18] provide useful frameworks to explore the different types of knowledge base required in palliative care. Each is important in its own right; however, they overlap, and are interrelated.

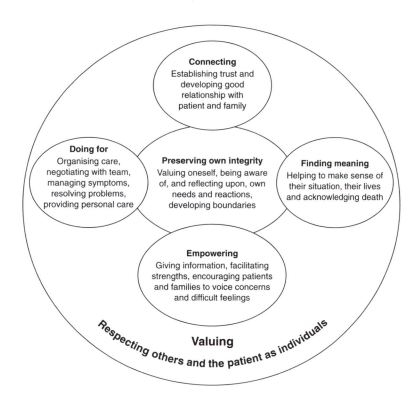

**Figure 1.1**  Dimensions of supportive role.[16]

---

**Box 1.1   Three kinds of knowing (Habermas)**[17]

1 *Instrumental/technical knowing* – acquisition of skills and understanding.
2 *Communicative knowing* – interpersonal relations, social and cultural under-standing.
3 *Emancipatory knowing* – self-understanding, awareness and transformation.

---

**Box 1.2   Four patterns of knowing (Carper)**[18]

1 *Empirics* – based on scientific evidence-based approach and can be seen as *know that* knowledge. This includes objective knowledge about the disease process, technical knowledge, symptom management and nursing inter-ventions based on an evidence base.
2 *Ethical* – awareness and understanding of ethical, moral and professional issues, notions of right or wrong. This area is integral in all decision making in palliative care and underpins our professional judgement.

3 *Personal* – based on gaining self-mastery, becoming self-aware and self-reflective. This personal knowing is at the heart of our ability to care for others and the development of a therapeutic relationship. We need to have compassion for ourselves; we need, as carers, to be our own carers first. If we can learn to sit with and understand our own pain, anger or fear, have compassion and forgive ourselves, then we are more likely to be there for the patient and his or her family.

4 *Aesthetic* – based on intuition and intuitive learning and is considered to be the art and *know how* of nursing. Intuition enables people to respond to things creatively using imagination and abstract thinking. It is this knowledge that enables us to have *an intuitive grasp*. We are able to know what to do. We know that something is right or recognise a change in someone's condition without consciously knowing why. When we try to describe aesthetic knowledge we often find ourselves lost for words. This can also be seen as tacit knowledge.

## Novice to expert

We need to evolve from being novice practitioners to expert practitioners. As novices, we need to be taught technical and rule-based knowledge and do things *by the book*. As experts, we need to be able to unconsciously utilise and incorporate all the above knowledge and develop our *'intuitive grasp'*. To be *expert*, we cannot solely rely on our art; we need to test out and challenge our theory-based knowledge in practice, and to systematically record and reflect upon our practice-based knowledge. Only through this can expertise be achieved. We develop expertise through:

- interpreting clinical situations
- exploring and critiquing the evidence
- making complex decisions.

Therefore, knowledge is embedded in clinical expertise.[19]

**Self-assessment exercise 1.1**
**Time: 30 minutes**

Consider how you might use:

- Davies and Oberle's aspects[16]
- Carper's ways of knowing[18]
- Benner's concept of novice to expert[19]

as a framework for caring for dying patients.

Identify:

- where you think you are on the novice–expert continuum
- what you know from theory and practice
- what your learning needs are.

Consider:

- how you learnt your knowledge
- how you might meet your learning needs.

# So how do we learn this knowledge?

The government, in its modernisation agenda,[20] has recognised lifelong learning. Continuing professional development (CPD) is imperative for all professionals to enable them to demonstrate their competence to practise. Importantly, formal and informal learning are recognised as of equal value. Learning from practice and experience is viewed as essential.

The introduction of the *Knowledge and Skills Framework* within *Agenda for Change*[21] will assist managers and practitioners in identifying competence and areas of need, and explicitly identifies ways in which learning needs can be met including:

- off-job learning and development with others
- on-job learning and development
- off-job learning and development on one's own.

Figure 1.2 provides a summary of what we need to consider and include when learning about palliative care.

## Off-job learning and development with others: classroom-based learning

Traditionally, learning has been seen as formal. Taking place in the classroom and during one's youth, it was seen as something the teacher did to a learner. Teachers, *who were more knowledgeable*, imparted information to *those who knew less*. This form of learning is derived from a didactic approach. Those advocating an experiential approach challenge this. They argue that for learning to take place, learners need to be active, and process, interpret and make sense of what is presented to them. These paradigms are not opposed to each other but are at opposite ends of the spectrum; both have their place. Traditional or didactic programmes highlight knowledge and information whereas experiential programmes encourage self-direction, reflection and involvement (*see* Box 1.3).[22]

---

**Box 1.3   Distinctions between the two kinds of learning**[23]

| *Significant experiential learning* | *Traditional conventional learning* |
|---|---|
| Personal involvement | Prescribed curriculum |
| Whole person | Similar for all students |
| Self-initiated | Lecturing |
| Pervasive | Standardised testing |
| Evaluated by learner | Instructor-evaluated |
| Essence is meaning | Essence is knowing and reproducing |

---

Despite the recognition of the effectiveness of an active experiential approach to learning,[24] the formal, more traditional didactic lecture style is still predominant in palliative care education and training, thus providing little opportunity for debate, discussion or personal sharing and learning.[25]

Adults need more self-directed learning, with the teacher being a guide and facilitator, utilising their expertise to stimulate learning rather than to communicate a body of knowledge.[23] The key is not so much to consider *what* you are learning but *how* you are learning. Even in traditional lecture sessions, you can

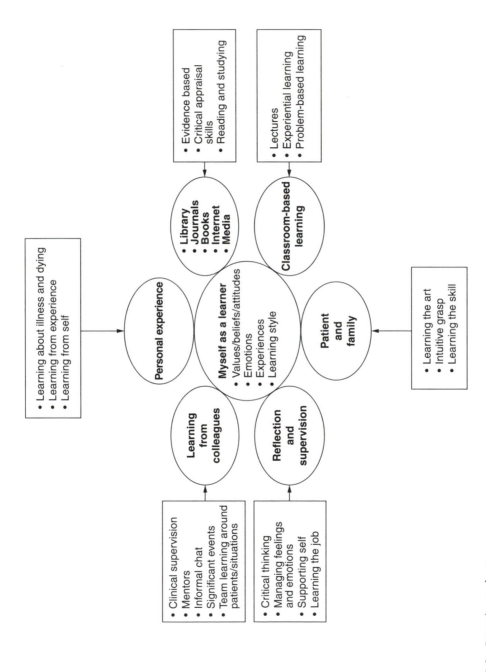

Figure 1.2   Learning to learn.

enhance your learning through questioning *what is being said* and relating it to *your own experience*, rather than just taking notes to be put aside once the lecture is over.

---

**Self-assessment exercise 1.2**
**Time: 10 minutes**

Think about the last palliative care course/study day you attended.

- What was the topic?
- Which model of learning was being used?

---

As learners in palliative care, you need to be aware and questioning of how you are taught. Are you:

- involved in the learning
- encouraged to reflect, process and apply knowledge to experience?

Learning symptom management is not the same as learning pharmacology; the lecture approach is not sufficient. It may provide you with information but will not assist you in applying it to practice.

Teaching approaches need to take into account the true complexity of symptom management of the terminally ill, considering all of the *domains of knowledge*.[18] Teaching strategies need to encompass three learning domains:

- *cognitive* – thinking, making sense, questioning (lecture, case studies)
- *affective* – exploring our attitudes and emotions (self-reflection)
- *psychomotor* – doing, skills development (learning through experience).[26]

Research demonstrates that the more we are involved in the learning process, the more we learn (*see* Figure 1.3), and gives credence to the old Chinese proverb:

- I hear and I forget
- I see and I remember
- I do and I understand.

The learning pyramid (Figure 1.3) further illustrates this point. Only 5% of information received from listening in a didactic session is likely to be retained, whereas when we are allowed to learn through 'doing', the retention rate goes up to 75%.

## Learning styles and whole-brain thinking

People have different learning styles[27,28] and are either right- or left-brain thinkers.[29] Left-brain thinking tends to be logical and systematic whereas right-brain thinking sees the big picture and is creative and intuitive. For learning to be effective, you will need to become confident with different learning styles and develop whole-brain thinking.

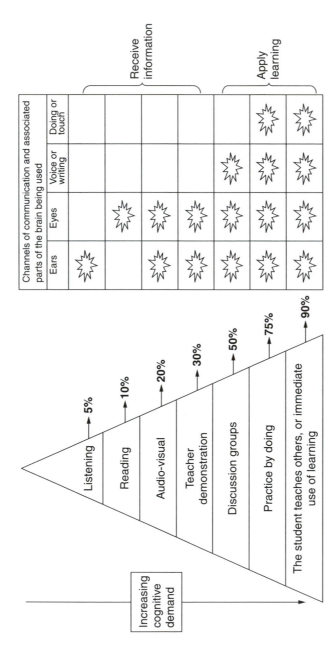

**Figure 1.3** The learning pyramid. *Source: Research on the recall rate of different learning activities. National Training Laboratories, Maine.*

> **Self-assessment exercise 1.3**
> **Time: 30 minutes**
>
> Look up Honey and Munford's *learning styles questionnaire.*[28]
>
> - Are you an activist, reflector, theorist or pragmatist?
> - Are you a right- or left-brain thinker – or both?

## Experiential learning

Experiential learning is the most effective form of learning in palliative care.[30-32] Experiential learning means learning from:

- current or past experience through sharing and reflecting upon your own experiences
- artificially created experiences; these may involve:
  - role-play
  - scenario-based learning
  - creative approaches.

Experiential learning requires you, as the learner, to place your whole self in the situation, to develop critical and self-awareness. This can be daunting for those unused to this form of learning, believing that they are there to learn – and the teacher is there to teach.

## Hearing the voice of the user

Have you attended an education and teaching session in which a patient or carer has recalled their story and shared what it is like to be ill, dying, and the recipient of healthcare? It helps to put ourselves in others' shoes, which can be very difficult when someone is angry or distressed. Although you work with patients every day, actually sitting down and hearing *how it is*, in a classroom situation, can be challenging and upsetting.

## Problem-based learning

A new experiential learning strategy in palliative care is *problem-based learning*. This student-centred approach provides a systematic interactive approach to critical thinking and clinical judgement combined with the use of reflective journals to encourage learners to reflect on, and learn from, practice. This approach provides:

- increased self-awareness
- more positive attitudes towards death
- enhanced communication in difficult situations
- emotional support
- critical thinking
- teamwork.[6]

This could be a valuable approach to interdisciplinary learning in palliative care, enabling and enhancing:

- a shared understanding of each other
- collaboration
- patient and family care.

## Learning to be a critical thinker

Critical thinking is an attitude and reasoning process involving a number of intellectual skills.[33] Critical thinking requires objective and subjective qualities. It requires the ability:

- to think rationally, logically, practically and theoretically
- to demonstrate self-awareness, creativity, sensitivity and responsiveness to others.

It requires:

- cognitive skills including decision making, problem-solving skills, intuition
- people to think independently, have intellectual humility, integrity, courage, empathy and perseverance
- people to distinguish intuition from prejudice.

To become a critical thinker you need to:

- critique evidence
- reflect on your experience
- question yourself, your behaviour, emotions, fears, responses, values, attitudes and assumptions.

You need to consider the impact of the wider political, social and economic context on palliative care. Consider power differences and imbalances, as well as ingrained rituals and practices, organisational and professional restraints, and the impact of the ward/practice culture. With an open mind you need to listen to:

- opposing views
- new ideas
- learning methods
- your own and others' feelings.

Most of all, you need to be prepared to unlearn what you think is right, and your own views about yourself.

## Learning about dying

Learning about caring for dying people is emotionally hard. As human beings, we have anxieties and fears about death, and may have had personal, as well as professional, experiences of death. We often feel we have failed dying people. Talking about dying can bring painful memories and emotions, particularly if you have felt unsupported at the time and have learnt to deal with these by *'being professional'* and moving on. Given these challenges, it is not surprising that groups can sometimes develop a momentum of their own, with individuals reacting negatively, disrupting or sabotaging the group. Experiential learning about dying, and for the group to develop *safety* and *trust*, needs careful negotiating and facilitation.[34]

Learning in the classroom is only a small part of our learning in palliative care. However, it is useful because it takes us out of the *comfort zone*, allowing us space to reflect, gain confidence and learn to think critically, having the opportunity to intensely explore all dimensions of palliative care knowledge.

## On-job learning and development: non-classroom-based learning

Learning is embedded in experience and practice. It is the heart of lifelong learning. Although recognised by professional bodies and the *Knowledge and Skills Framework*, it is currently easier to be released for a study day than to be given time to learn in and from practice. Aesthetic knowledge hinges on this form of learning. If you are motivated to evolve from novice to expert then you may have to be proactive and challenge this.

### Learning to manage feelings and emotions

Although emotional labour is an essential part of palliative care,[35] it is an area until recently neglected in the curriculum. People develop their own coping strategies and often learn to distance themselves from difficult or painful situations,[36] thus affecting their relationship with patients. Often the person in charge sets the emotional climate. Crying or showing emotions is not deemed professional. If people are nurtured and supported, they are more likely to be able to give openly to others, to develop appropriate boundaries and avoid burnout.[37]

Mentors and peers are helpful in enabling professionals learn this skill. Knowing they have an opportunity to be heard, the professional learns to suppress the distress until s/he finds a suitable moment to grieve.[38] Through increased self-awareness s/he learns to create a form of professional membrane, retaining sensitivity to patients while retaining integrity: able to be present but not enmeshed.[38]

Patients and families may remind us of people we know, challenge us emotionally, and/or cause us to be angry or upset. It is not easy to be honest about negative feelings. However, it is impossible to be completely non-judgemental; some people will inevitably push our buttons. To develop self-awareness it is important to look at your emotions and reactions to people.

---

**Self-assessment exercise 1.4**
**Time: 15 minutes**

Consider:

- how you manage your emotions
- how you learnt to do this
- what are your coping strategies
- who presses your buttons?

---

## Learning from mentors

Mentorship and shadowing are recognised as essential in the education and training of students and the support of preceptors but are rarely used in day-to-day practice. Consider finding yourself someone who is knowledgeable and experienced in palliative care whom you can spend time with in practice. Identify someone with good interpersonal skills that you trust and respect. Invite them to be your mentor, to help you reflect and learn from your practice and share your emotional pain. They will need to be able to befriend, support, challenge, confront, question and coach you and to commit to a regular period. Agree ground rules, learning objectives and a review date. Begin each session with a reflection on an incident, and then explore new understanding. Finally, develop an action plan. Use a reflective model or framework if you find them helpful.

## Learning with a peer

Identify a colleague with whom you feel you can have an equal, reciprocal relationship. Invite them to act as peer support. You will both need all the qualities of a mentor. You can establish the relationship in a similar way. You may find it easier to be honest with each other but be less willing to challenge and analyse.

## Reflection on practice

People often 'do' reflective practice on a course and then stop. If you are inexperienced in reflection, it can help to use a model or cycle. Do this with a peer or mentor before sharing it with a group.[39,40] Reflect on an incident or situation, or keep a reflective journal. Developing your reflective skills takes time, practice and patience; the more you do, the more expert you become. It enables you to:

- identify what happened
- note ritualistic care
- reflect on your evidence base
- explore your strengths and your feelings
- be clearer about what you have learnt and what you might do differently in the future.

Moreover, it helps to identify learning in practice, the value of colleagues and learning from patients and carers.

---

**Self-assessment exercise 1.5**
**Time: 15 minutes**

- Have you ever experienced an intuitive grasp?
- Identify an example and write about it.

Using what, how, when and whom:

- Describe the situation.
- Explain why you think it was an intuitive grasp.
- Was it accurate?
- How would you explain the phenomenon now?

## Learning from significant events/critical incidents: *interdisciplinary learning*

Significant event analysis is a routine part of primary care. Teams meet together and reflect upon a patient or a situation. This can be an experience that went well, or one that presented a challenge.

In challenging ongoing situations, all professionals involved in the situation should:

- meet regularly
- share information, personal reactions and experiences
- discuss care options.

This facilitates realisation that others experience similar difficulties – that they are not alone in their distress. It enables a greater understanding of individual roles and encourages shared learning. *Try to establish these within your own workplace.*

## Learning through keeping a reflective journal

> *The journal is a space, like an eddy within a fast moving stream, where I can pause from the often hectic and reactive effort of stream life in order to reflect and see things the way they are.*[40]

Story telling and journal writing are useful learning techniques in palliative care and facilitate the discovery of practice-based knowledge.[40,41]

You may want to use a reflective cycle, cues or even to consider creative expression. Often we feel inadequate when it comes to creativity. However, we are limited only by our own conditioning, imagination and motivation. You may wish to paint a picture and see what happens, or, following a death, write a poem; let it wander until it tells you how you feel. Perhaps you could sing a song you create yourself. Try free writing, where you just begin to write and see what happens. This can enable you to capture the richness and beauty of practice when sometimes it all feels too much. Write about incidents or practice within 24 hours to recapture the whole situation. Begin with writing down negative feelings. Writing it down also helps to 'let it go' – for example, 'I feel angry because ... or I am so sad because ...'[40]

Show parts of your journal to people you trust; they will help you explore deeper, and not only to challenge your attitudes and practice, but validate them. However, it takes courage do this – to be self-critical, acknowledge our mistakes and admit that we are not always caring and that, sometimes, it is difficult to cope.

---

**Self-assessment exercise 1.6**
**Time: 20 minutes**

Choose a recent incident, try some form of creative expression, and see what happens.

---

## Learning from patients and carers

The patient and family are our biggest learning resource. Each person, if we listen, can teach us something about the experience of being ill, our assumptions and ourselves. Furthermore, each of us has some personal experience of being a patient, a family member and/or of bereavement. Instead of setting this to one side, reflect on this; explore what we have learnt from being on the receiving end.

### Off-job learning and development on one's own

Consider looking at other learning resources such as:

• videos
• media
• internet
• intranet
• computer-assisted learning packages
• e-learning programmes.

Regularly read journals, utilise books within your library and identify a particular topic or project to undertake.

---

**Self-assessment exercise 1.7**
**Time: 1 hour**

Identify a patient or family member who you think taught you a lot.

• What did you learn? This could be your experience as a patient, family member or someone you have cared for.
• With permission, interview a patient or carer about their experience.

---

## Conclusion

One of our greatest challenges in learning palliative care is death and dying. We care for dying people in a society in which death has become increasingly taboo. It is no longer seen as an acceptable and natural part of living.[42] Professionals experience considerable death anxieties. It is inevitable that we will find it difficult to confront the reality of death.[13] Learning to be an expert in palliative care is, therefore, challenging and, like living, is a lifelong endeavour. We need to develop a blended learning approach that incorporates learning from our own experiences, practice, classroom and other learning resources.

It is hoped that this chapter has helped you to consider the breadth of knowledge necessary, and ways in which you may learn. *Most important of all is your need to learn to know, value and care for yourself.*

---

**Post-reading exercise 1.1**
**Time: 15 minutes**

• Identify your learning needs.
• Develop your personal learning action plan.

Ensure you identify the most appropriate ways of learning to meet your needs. What about:

- a secondment
- a mentor
- shadowing
- a reflective journal
- team learning
- other?

## References

1   Buckley J. Holism and a health promoting approach to palliative care. *Int J Palliative Nursing*. 2002; **8**: 505–508.
2   Field D. Palliative medicine and the medicalisation of death. *European Journal of Cancer Care*. 1994; **3**: 58–62.
3   Quint JC. *The Nurse and the Dying Patient*. New York: Macmillan; 1967.
4   Whitfield S. *A Descriptive Study of Student Nurses' Ward Experiences with Dying Patients and Their Attitudes Towards Them*. Unpublished MSc thesis. Manchester: University of Manchester; 1979.
5   Field D. Formal instruction in United Kingdom medical schools about death and dying. *Medical Education*. 1984; **18**: 429–434.
6   Mok E, Man LW, Wong FK. The issue of death and dying: employing problem based learning in nursing education. *Nurse Education Today*. 2002; **22**: 319–329.
7   Twycross R, Lack SA. *Symptom Control in Far-advanced Cancer: pain relief*. London: Pitman; 1983.
8   Addington-Hall J. *Reaching Out: specialist palliative care for adults with non-malignant disease*. Occasional Paper 14. London: National Council for Hospice and Specialist Palliative Care Services; 1998.
9   Corner J, Wilson-Barrett J. The newly registered nurse and the cancer patient: an educational evaluation. *International Journal of Palliative Nursing Studies*. 1992; **29**(2): 177–190.
10  Beck CT. Nursing students' experiences caring for dying patients. *Journal of Nursing Education*. 1997; **36**(9): 408–415.
11  Hafferty FW. *Into the Valley: death and the socialisation of medical students*. New Haven: Yale University Press; 1991.
12  Yates P, Clinton M, Hart G. Improving psychosocial care: a professional development programme. *International Journal of Palliative Nursing*. 1996; **2**(4): 212–216.
13  Copp G. Palliative nursing education: a review of the research findings. *Journal of Advanced Nursing*. 1994; **19**: 552–557.
14  National Institute for Health and Clinical Excellence (NICE). *Guidance on Cancer Services: improving supportive and palliative care for adults with cancer. The manual*. London: NICE; 2004.
15  James C, Macleod R. The problematic nature of education in palliative care. *Journal of Palliative Care*. 1993; **9**(4): 5–10.
16  Davies B, Oberle K. Dimensions of the supportive role of the nurse in palliative care. *Oncology Nursing Forum*. 1990; **17**(1): 87–94.
17  Habermas J. *Knowledge and Human Interest*. London: Heinemann; 1978.
18  Carper BA. Fundamental patterns of knowing in nursing. *Advances in Nursing Science*. 1978; **1**(1): 13–23.
19  Benner P. *From Novice to Expert: excellence and power in clinical practice*. Menlo Park, California: Addison Wesley; 1984.
20  Department of Health. *A First Class Service Quality Service in the New NHS*. London: Department of Health Publications; 1998.
21  Department of Health. *The NHS Knowledge and Skills Framework (NHS KSF) and the Development Review Process*. London: Department of Health Publishing; 2004. http://www.dh.gov.uk/assetRoot/04/09/08/61/04090861.pdf

22 Rogers CR. *Freedom to Learn for the 80s*. Columbus, OH: Merrill; 1983.

23 Rogers A. *Teaching Adults*, 3rd edition. Maidenhead: Open University Publications; 2002.

24 Hurtig WA, Stewin L. The effect of death education and experience on nursing students' attitude towards death. *Journal of Advanced Nursing*. 1990; 15(1): 29–34.

25 Becker R. Education in cancer and palliative care: an international perspective. In: Foyle L, Hostad J, editors. *Delivering Cancer and Palliative Care Education*. Oxford: Radcliffe Medical Press; 2004.

26 Bloom BS. *Taxonomy of Educational Objectives*. London: Longman; 1965.

27 Kolb DA. *Learning Style Inventory Technical Manual*. Boston, MA: McBer; 1976.

28 Honey P, Mumford A. *Manual of Learning Styles*, revised edition. London: Peter Honey; 1992.

29 Sperry R, Ornstein R. In: Rose C, editor. *Accelerated Learning*, 4th edition. Buckingham: Accelerated Learning Publications; 1989.

30 Wilkinson S, Bailey K, Aldridge J *et al*. A longitudinal evaluation of a communication skills programme. *Palliative Medicine*. 1999; 13: 341–348.

31 Maguire P, Booth K, Elliott C *et al*. Helping health professionals involved in cancer care acquire key interviewing skills – the impact of workshops. *Eur J of Cancer*. 1996; 32: 1486–1489.

32 Durlak JA, Reisenberg LA. The impact of death education. *Death Studies*. 1991; 15: 39–58.

33 Wilkinson JM. *Nursing Process – a critical thinking approach*. Menlo Park, California: Eddison-Wesley Nursing; 1996.

34 Spall R, Johnson M. Experiential exercises in palliative care training. *International J of Palliative Nursing*. 1997; 3(4): 222–226.

35 James N. Emotional labour. *Sociological Review*. 1989; 37: 15–42.

36 Wilkinson S. Factors which influence how nurses communicate with cancer patients. *Journal of Advanced Nursing*. 1991; 16(6): 677–688.

37 Smith P, Gray B. Reassessing the concept of emotional labour in student nurse education: role of link lecturers and mentors in a time of change. *Nurse Education Today*. 2001; 21: 230–237.

38 Spouse J. *Professional Learning in Nursing*. Oxford: Blackwell; 2003.

39 Gibbs G. *Learning by Doing: a guide to teaching and learning methods*. Oxford: Further Education Unit, Oxford Brooks University; 1988.

40 Johns C. *Being Mindful, Easing Suffering: reflections on palliative care*. London: Jessica Kingsley; 2004.

41 Attig T. Person centred death education. *Death Studies*. 1992; 16: 357–370.

42 Becker E. *The Denial of Death*. New York: Free Press; 1973.

# To learn more

## Books

- Foyle L, Hostad J, editors. *Delivering Cancer and Palliative Care Education*. Oxford: Radcliffe Medical Press; 2004.
- Jeffrey D, editor. *Teaching Palliative Care: a practical guide*. Oxford: Radcliffe Medical Press; 2002.
- Souse J. *Professional Learning in Nursing*. Oxford: Blackwell; 2003.

## Websites

- www.dipex.org
- www.helpthehospices.org.uk/elearning
- www.hospicecare.com
- www.hospiceinformation.info
- www.macmillan.org.uk
- www.mapfoundation.org
- www.nelh.nhs.uk
- www.rosettalife.org

# Complementary chapters

*See also Stepping into Palliative Care 1: relationships and responses*

- Chapter 2: What is palliative care?
- Chapter 3: The cancer journey
- Chapter 5: The psychological impact of serious illness
- Chapter 6: Hope and coping strategies
- Chapter 7: The therapeutic relationship
- Chapter 10: Understanding the needs of the palliative care team
- Chapter 11: The value of teamwork
- Chapter 12: Stress issues in palliative care
- Chapter 13: Communication: the essence of good practice, management and leadership.

*See also Stepping into Palliative Care 2: care and practice*

- Chapter 12: Hearing the pain of the carer
- Chapter 13: Spirituality and palliative care
- Chapter 14: Bereavement

# Chapter 2

# What is palliative care?

*Vicky Robinson*

---

**Pre-reading exercise 2.1**
**Time: 10 minutes**

- Spend a few moments thinking why you want to read this chapter.
- Can you recall a patient who died leaving you feeling that you could or should have done more to ease their pain?
- Keep this person in mind as you read this chapter.

---

*You matter because you are you. You matter to the last moment of your life, and we will do all we can to help you not only to die peacefully, but also to live until you die.*[1]

This quote captures the essence of the work of Dame Cicely Saunders, founder of the modern hospice movement, who died in July 2005 at St Christopher's – the hospice she founded in South East London. She dedicated her life to the care of the dying and was a qualified nurse, social worker and doctor. Dame Cicely brought together the importance of sound research and good education as being essential components of skilled and compassionate care of the dying. Her early work was in the efficacy of morphine. This concept of the regular pre-emptive approach to pain control was revolutionary and changed the fate of dying people.

In theory, and to a degree in practice, end-of-life care has come a long way since those early days, and palliative care is now a familiar term in healthcare. In 1987 it became a recognised medical specialty. But what does it really mean to those working in health and social care in the 21st century? This chapter focuses on three areas.

1 *Palliative care – the speciality*: the history of the modern hospice movement and the beginnings of palliative care in the NHS provide a context in which we can begin to understand the nature and purpose of end-of-life care.
2 *The art of palliative care – making and maintaining relationships*: how we can engage individuals and families and help them to face an uncertain future.
3 *Becoming a resilient practitioner*: we look briefly at how we as professionals can develop resilience and '*not grow weary of doing good*',[2] in this hard, sad, but by no means hopeless area of healthcare.

# Palliative care – the speciality

The word *palliative* is derived from the Latin verb *palliare*, which means *to cloak* or *to hide*.

The World Health Organization (WHO) defined palliative care as follows:[3]

> *Palliative care ... is an approach that improves the quality of life of patients and their families facing the problems associated with life threatening illness, through the **prevention and the relief of suffering** by means of early identification and impeccable assessment and treatment of pain and other problems, physical, psychosocial and spiritual:*
> - *affirms life and regards dying as a normal process*
> - *provides relief from pain and other symptoms*
> - *intends neither to hasten nor postpone death*
> - *integrates psychological and spiritual aspects of care*
> - *offers a support system to help patients to live as actively as possible until death*
> - *offers a support system to help the family cope during the patient's illness and in their own bereavement*
> - *uses a team approach to address the needs of patients and families, including bereavement counselling if indicated*
> - *enhances the quality of life, and may also positively influence the course of illness*
> - *is applicable early in the course of the illness, in conjunction with other therapies that are intended to prolong life, such as chemotherapy or radiation therapy, and includes those investigations needed to better understand and manage distressing clinical complications.*[3]

While the history of palliative care, and in particular the modern hospice movement, is rooted in cancer care at the end of life, it is now recognised that the principles of hospice care are applicable to all life-threatening illnesses, and not only in the dying phase.

Doctors undertaking specialist training in palliative medicine are required to attain competencies in areas other than the pure science of pain and symptom management. In nursing, there are palliative care competencies published by the Royal College of Nursing and Marie Curie Cancer Care. Recently, St Christopher's Hospice has introduced competencies for nurses working in specialist palliative care[4] in line with the National Health Service (NHS) Knowledge and Skills Framework.

## The history of palliative care

Figure 2.1 demonstrates the advances of the palliative care movement.

### Landscape 1: the first frontier – laying the foundations

This came with the establishment of the modern hospice movement and Cicely Saunders' early research on the use of morphine in the relief of cancer pain.[5] Her seminal work laid the foundations for the establishment of a range of therapeutics for pain and symptom relief at the end of life. Saunders' work did not end here. Being a qualified nurse and social worker caused her to place equal emphasis on the psychosocial and spiritual care of a person and their loved ones: in other words, care

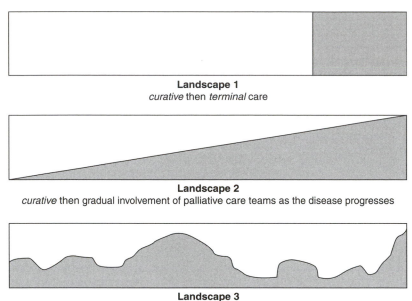

**Landscape 1**
*curative* then *terminal* care

**Landscape 2**
*curative* then gradual involvement of palliative care teams as the disease progresses

**Landscape 3**
palliative care approach in conjunction with *curative* treatments

**Figure 2.1** The landscape of palliation.

of the whole person. The notion of total pain[6] at the end of life became the signature of the modern hospice movement. In the UK 220 hospices provide this type of care.[7]

## Landscape 2: the second frontier – spreading the word

As hospices continued to develop, community teams based in hospices offered support at home. The early 1980s heralded the establishment of teams in the NHS. Major cancer charities (e.g. Macmillan Cancer Support,[8] Marie Curie Cancer Care[9]) began funding palliative care posts and services to work in the NHS and charitable sector. Largely based in hospitals they provided advice and support to patients and professionals. Because they were *on site*, there were opportunities for the teams to work alongside oncologists and other specialists in providing support and information as the patient began to deteriorate.[10] Many of these teams reached out to the community, using the hospice model to offer support at home to patients and families, general practitioners and community nurses.

## The HIV phenomenon – a new approach?

The emergence of HIV (human immunodeficiency virus) in the 1980s posed some fundamental challenges which moved the speciality to its next stage:

- *first* – how to cope with the young dying, many of whom were from a gay lifestyle, or were drug users
- *second* – many patients continued with *curative* treatments to the point of death

- *third* – the symptom burden of HIV included problems not hitherto presented in palliative care (e.g. profuse diarrhoea, encephalopathic illnesses, severe and intractable infections).

Suddenly palliative care was not a discrete area of clinical practice reserved for hospice care and hospital support teams, nearly all of whom dealt only with cancer. The answer was to take the hospice model, adapt it and apply it to times of crisis when the issue for the patient is an uncertain future of having to adapt to periods of acute illness with the possibility of death or remission/recovery.[11,12]

Figure 2.2 shows two disease trajectories that were familiar to practitioners involved in cancer and HIV care in the 1990s. In the HIV population, the disease was so uncertain and the symptoms so severe and unpredictable that it was normal practice for palliative care to be involved intermittently throughout a disease journey, whereas in cancer there was still the tendency to refer on to palliative care once curative treatment had ended.

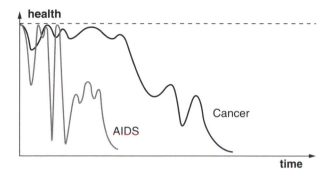

**Figure 2.2**  Two types of disease trajectory.

Alongside this, isolated services were looking seriously at all diagnoses that may be in need of palliation and beginning to develop and adapt the philosophy of palliative care accordingly with the coining of two phrases: generic palliative care and *the disadvantaged dying*.[13,14]

## Landscape 3: the final frontier – palliative care for all

There are now 358 specialist community teams and 293 hospital support teams in the UK. The last 10 years have brought projects such as the Liverpool Care Pathway (integrated care pathway), the Gold Standards Framework and the Preferred Place of Care, all of which are designed to improve palliative care across the country. In March 2004, the National Institute for Clinical Excellence (NICE) released its *Guidance for Supportive and Palliative Care for Adults with Cancer.*[15]

Palliative care for non-cancer is being promoted in government documents.[16–18] Various charities are funding palliative care nursing posts[19,20] dedicated to diseases other than cancer.

Having looked at the definition of palliative care and how services have developed over the last 50 years, we turn now to the nature and purpose of palliative care in relation to the people in our care.

# The art of palliative care – making and maintaining relationships

What is palliative care? In a nutshell, it is the management of suffering through understanding what it is for each person, how to break it into manageable chunks and then how to overcome it. This is not easy. It is a task that requires a view of the person as a whole, and several disciplines working as a team with the patient and family. The starting point has to be the making and maintaining of relationships with patients, their families and colleagues.

## '... through the prevention and relief of suffering ...'[3]

Pharmacological and non-pharmacological approaches to pain and symptom management are dealt with in other chapters but we need to understand that pain and symptom management are not ends in themselves; *they are there merely to palliate* (that is, provide a cloak for) *the disease process so that the patient has the space to make decisions and conclude their life as meaningfully as possible.* How can *we* help?

In recent years the emphasis has been on the relief of pain and physical symptoms. But a mechanistic approach to this cannot address issues of meaning, and how a patient and family may present to us. Let us turn to the manifestation and management of non-physical pain and symptoms, in other words *suffering*. The simple model in Figure 2.3 offers a framework through which to work. In three parts, it helps us to examine another's world through its layers to the core. It is a model developed some years ago and recently published elsewhere.[21]

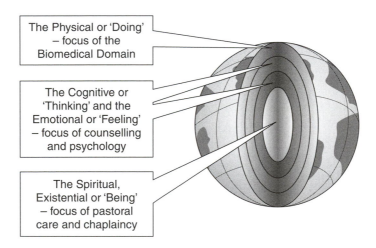

The Physical or 'Doing' – focus of the Biomedical Domain

The Cognitive or 'Thinking' and the Emotional or 'Feeling' – focus of counselling and psychology

The Spiritual, Existential or 'Being' – focus of pastoral care and chaplaincy

**Figure 2.3** The schematic layers within our world relevant to suffering.

## The outer layer: the physical or 'doing' domain

Physical health, agility and ability to achieve provide us with great protection of what lies beneath the surface of our lives. Therefore, illness can leave us exposed to unfamiliar or long-buried insecurities. We all will recall times in our own or others' lives when physical illness such as flu or a stomach upset has prevented us from doing something important, and how that can leave us feeling. Most of us are *human doings* rather than human beings. Towards the end of life, physical deterioration can provide the professional with the entrée through which one may begin to expose the deeper meanings and fears that will surface with disability, deterioration and dying. Nurses and doctors in particular have these privileges and it is vital that we do not stop at prescribing medication or undertaking a nursing task. Patients will describe real practical problems as their body deteriorates. As well as offering practical solutions, probing to gain a deeper understanding of what the impact is for that individual, and their loved ones, will almost invariably result in a deepening trust and growth in the therapeutic relationship.

Many patients, families and professionals will describe feelings of helplessness. What people usually mean is that they feel they are no longer in control of their lives. Our lives are largely centred on the ability to achieve (money, fame, success, physical beauty). Patients often feel robbed of their independence, status and privacy, areas we all cherish – our so-called *safe places*. Knowing you are going to die means that these safe places are no longer there. We have to find a way to turn a human *doing* into a human *being*.

## The middle layer: the psychological, social, emotional and 'feeling' domain

This domain, when suffering exists, can move us deeper into the person and may expose the underlying meanings about thoughts, emotions and behaviours. While there may be some overlap with mental health, this source of suffering is distinct from a defined mental illness (a biomedical diagnosis). Within this *feeling* domain patients and families may express any of the following concerns.

- How to live with the emotional impact and strain of practical or financial pressures.
- Feeling emotionally up and down – it is important to try to understand how the patient is feeling *now* as opposed to how they want to feel; what the triggers are to feelings; how this manifests, for example:
  - How are the symptoms (physical or otherwise) affecting the patient and those around them and how in turn are these fed back to the patient?
  - Does the patient trust us to deal effectively with these symptoms both now and in the future?
  - If the patient's mood is flat, are they simply reacting appropriately to their situation or is there a depressive element?
- How to deal with their important emotional relationships – in working with patients and families at the end of life it is important to understand how and to whom the patient relates to the people and the world around them. Genograms (family trees) are extremely useful as they can be completed by the professional and patient together. These can show diagrammatically the family history and relationships with relatives, friends and others (e.g. colleagues). This may help us uncover the relationships that need some attention or facilitation:
  - *broken* relationships may be those close to the patient, within their immediate circle of family or friends, or they may be more distant, in terms of both space and time
  - *dead* relationships are essential to explore, and yet are the most frequently neglected. This includes relationships with people who are deceased, most

commonly parents, but not infrequently children or grandchildren. More difficult are relationships with people who are still alive, such as divorced spouses or family estrangements or feuds.

- Those who have lived through human conflict will have wounds deeply buried. Among the elderly, World War II still casts its shadow and through globalisation professionals are encountering many more patients who are refugees. Refugees and survivors of wars are increasingly presenting with disease and suffering, though their needs are specialised.

These areas of psychological, social and emotional suffering can be helped greatly given the right expertise, approach and motivation by the patient. However, the work may be time consuming and might need specialist help. Nevertheless, *if we do not look, we will not uncover these remediable areas.*

## The core: the spiritual/existential domain

*As a society we are very bad at talking about death ...*[22]

The spiritual and existential or *ontological* (the way in which we see the nature of our being which includes beyond death) encompasses the fundamental questions of life and death. Therefore, it is seen as central to any person's identity/ontology and the conscious or unconscious river to their values, motivations and ethos. Some patients may not wish to address these questions explicitly but unresolved issues of belief may still underlie the intensity of the suffering arising in the *feeling* and *doing* domains. Even the strongest beliefs are stretched to the full as death approaches.

We will all face the inevitability and irreversibility of death at some stage in our lives. Most of us put off addressing this until absolutely necessary. This means that many patients will face death for the first time, having lived their lives largely based in the *doing* and *feeling* domains. People often revisit their spiritual or religious roots. Guilt and bitterness associated with past experiences of religious practice often re-emerge at this time. Others will find sources of comfort.

Patients and families often ask:

- What it has all been about?
- Is there a meaning to my life?
- How does it fit into the big picture?
- Have I made a difference?
- Will I be remembered?
- What happens next?

### Arthur's story

---

**Case scenario 2.1**

Steve was a nurse with a specialist palliative care team. He had been visiting Arthur, an 80-year-old widower and war veteran, for a few weeks and had built up a rapport with him as they supported rival football teams. Arthur lived with his daughter. Steve knew they were a Catholic family, but Arthur did not like to discuss his own beliefs. As Arthur became weaker, he became withdrawn and depressed. He did not respond to antidepressants. Steve asked him if he would like to see a priest. Arthur said that he hadn't bothered with 'that stuff' and was 'not going to start now'. Steve returned to the office, feeling guilty as he thought he had 'intruded' or violated Arthur's integrity. A day or so later, Arthur's daughter rang to say that Arthur wanted to see Steve, but would not tell him why. Steve visited and Arthur told him his wartime story. He had been part of the British army that had liberated a large 'Nazi concentration camp'. Steve visited daily for the next 3 days and Arthur took great care to describe what he had seen, and what he had done, in minute detail. Never before had Arthur spoken to anyone of his wartime activities, and each day more detail of the atrocities that Arthur had seen unfolded. He spoke of his anger at what he had witnessed and his guilt at what he had done in response to this. Having 'tested' Steve's response, Arthur then agreed to see his local priest to receive absolution. He died peacefully within days.

Some, like Arthur, will find resolution in spiritual beliefs. Others will find resolution through understanding that they have made a difference, had loving relationships, procreated, led successful lives. There will be some patients who will resolve these areas privately. Patients may report dreams and hallucinations. These at times are not simply the side effects of medication. They can be the subconscious emerging and might require help from someone trained in work with the imagination and subconscious.

## Becoming a resilient practitioner

Caring for the dying patient and family is costly. Those who have been practising for many years have had to learn to move away from our identities as professional *human doings* to professional *human beings*. To be an effective practitioner requires a willingness to enter into a relationship with the patient that goes beyond the doing to/for towards the *being with* as people struggle to make sense of their lives and come to terms with death. The emotional impact of palliative care on the practitioner has been written about elsewhere[23] as has the importance of teamwork,[24] and how grief impacts the professional.[25]

In such situations, it can be common to refer on to the chaplaincy,[26] to deflect difficult questions by changing the subject (or *doing* something), or, at times, to become offended,[27] as one hides behind political correctness, and in some, as in Steve's case, to move out of the speciality. Steve left the speciality within months of Arthur's death. Steve was an effective and skilled communicator who gained trust from patients, families and colleagues alike. Steve had a great interest in philosophy and debate, but was unable to find meaning in the pain and suffering of his patients. During his leaving interview Steve said: '*I am unable to give any more of myself ... the work has made me very sad.*' This was despite regular clinical supervision, a stable home life and a supportive team environment. This need not be the case.

## Conclusion

I hope you have been encouraged to reflect on your views of palliative care, and possibly look at your beliefs about death and dying. *There are no secret answers to questions of pain and suffering – the answer is in the not knowing!* Medication assists with pain and symptom relief, colleagues and teams help with managing the processes, but in the intimate and privileged moments we have with the patient and family, *all we have is ourselves, our professional skills, experiences, and commitment to ensure that patients 'matter to the last moment of their lives'.*

## References

1 Saunders C. Care of the dying – 1 the problem of euthanasia. *Nursing Times.* 1976; 1 July: 1003–1005.
2 *Holy Bible.* 2 Thessalonians 3:13.
3 World Health Organization. *Definition of Palliative Care.* Geneva: WHO; 1990.
4 St Christopher's Hospice. *Competencies for Nurses: 'Making and maintaining relationships'.* 2005. available from Rae Keeley, St Christopher's Hospice. Email: r.keeley@stchristophers.org.uk.
5 Saunders C. Dying of cancer. *St Thomas's Hospital Gazette.* 1958; **56**(2): 37–47.
6 Saunders C. The philosophy of terminal care. In: Saunders C, editor. *The Management of Terminal Malignant Disease.* Baltimore MD: Arnold Publishers; 1984, pp. 232–241.
7 Help the Hospices. *Hospice Information: hospice and palliative care directory – United Kingdom and Ireland.* London: Help the Hospices; 2005.
8 Macmillan Cancer Support: www.macmillan.org.uk.
9 Marie Curie Cancer Care: www.mariecurie.org.uk.
10 Dunlop RJ, Hockley JM, editors. *Hospital-based Palliative Care Teams,* 2nd edition. Oxford: Oxford University Press; 1998.
11 George RJD. AIDS care team. *British Journal of Hospital Medicine.* 1989; **41**(1): 11.
12 George RJD. Palliation in AIDS – where do we draw the line? *Genitourinary Medicine.* 1991; April. **67**(2): 85–86.
13 Wasson K, George RJD. Non-cancer palliative care: the ethical argument in non-cancer palliative care. In: Higginson I, Addington-Hall J, editors. *Palliative Care for Non-Cancer Patients.* Oxford: Oxford University Press; 2001.
14 George RJD, Sykes J. Beyond cancer? In: Clark D, Ahmedzai S, Hockley J, editors. *New Themes in Palliative Care.* Oxford: Oxford University Press; 1997, pp. 239–254.
15 NICE: www.nice.org.uk.
16 Department of Health. *National Service Framework for Older People.* London: Department of Health Publications; 2001.
17 Department of Health. *National Service Framework for Coronary Heart Disease.* London: Department of Health Publications; 2000.
18 Department of Health. *National Service Framework for Long-term Conditions.* London: Department of Health Publications; 2005.
19 British Heart Foundation: www.bhf.org.uk.
20 Multiple Sclerosis Society: www.mssociety.org.uk.
21 George RJD, Martin J. Non-physical pain: suffering in action. In: Miles A, Finlay I, editors. *The Effective Management of Cancer Pain. UK key advances in clinical practice series,* 3rd edition. London: Aesculapius Press; 2003.
22 Cayton H. National Director for Patients and the Public. Part of speech made at launch of the King's Fund Care Project with South East London NHS Direct. October 2005.
23 Monroe B. The emotional impact of palliative care on staff. In: Sykes N, Edmonds P, Wiles J, editors. *Management of Advanced Disease,* 4th edition. London: Arnold; 2004.
24 Robinson V, George R. Teamworking. In: Sykes N, Fallon MT, Patt RB, editors. *Cancer Pain.* London: Arnold; 2003, pp. 95–104.
25 Papadatou D. A proposed model of health care professionals' grieving process. *Omega.* 2000; **41**(1): 59–77.

26   Ross LA. Spiritual aspects of nursing. *Journal of Advanced Nursing*. 1994; **19**: 439–447.
27   Walter T. Spirituality in palliative care: opportunity or burden? *Palliative Medicine*. 2002; **16**(2): 133–139.

## To learn more

- Becker R, Gamlin R. *Fundamental Aspects of Palliative Care Nursing*. Salisbury: MA Healthcare Ltd; 2004.
- O'Connor M, Aranda S, editors. *Palliative Care Nursing: a guide to practice*. Melbourne: Ausmed Publications; 2003.
- Payne S, Seymour J, Ingleton C, editors. *Palliative Care Nursing*. Milton Keynes: Open University Press; 2004.

## Complementary chapters

*See also Stepping into Palliative Care 1: relationships and responses*

- Chapter 3: The cancer journey
- Chapter 4: The experience of illness
- Chapter 5: The psychological impact of serious illness
- Chapter 7: The therapeutic relationship
- Chapter 8: Gold Standards Framework: a programme for community palliative care
- Chapter 9: Integrated care pathways
- Chapter 11: The value of teamwork
- Chapter 12: Stress issues in palliative care
- Chapter 15: Transcultural and ethnic issues at the end of life
- Chapter 16: Sexuality and palliative care

*See also Stepping into Palliative Care 2: care and practice*

- Chapter 1: Assessment in palliative care
- Chapter 13: Spirituality and palliative care

# Chapter 3

# The cancer journey

*Sheila Cassidy*

## Introduction

> **Pre-reading exercise 3.1**
> **Time: 10 minutes**
>
> Think about and list the different stages and encounters with health professionals experienced by a cancer patient during his or her '*journey*' from suspicion of cancer through to diagnosis and treatment to recovery or relapse and death.

The *cancer journey* is the experience of the patient with cancer, starting with suspicion of having something wrong through to diagnosis and treatment to recovery or relapse and death. It is made up of *encounters* with different professionals, which may be helpful, unhelpful or positively harmful. In between these *encounters* are the *intervals*: the time the patient has to wait, worry and speculate before the next stage of their journey. An example of an *interval* is the waiting between undergoing an investigation and receiving the results. The wheels of hospital administration often grind slowly, extending the period of waiting longer than is perhaps necessary and prolonging what can be an agony of worry, during which sleep is disrupted and tempers become daily more frayed.

My focus in this chapter is mainly on the *encounters*, rather than the *intervals*, because the quality of the former has a major effect upon the latter, i.e. if a professional is cool or brusque the patient is likely to feel put down and unhappy, whereas a little kindness and understanding go a long way to making the illness experience tolerable.

## The first encounter

The *first encounter* is with the suspicion that something is seriously wrong. An example of this is a woman who finds a lump in her breast or a man who suddenly passes blood in his urine or stool. Some people are not unduly alarmed, attributing rectal bleeding to piles, or a lump in the neck to a cyst. However, others instantly suspect cancer and react accordingly, thinking, '*Oh my God! I've got cancer, I'm going to die!*' At this *first encounter*, few, if any, people react logically. No woman thinks, '*Oh, I've got breast cancer but with modern treatment I'm sure I'll be fine.*' No – the discovery of a breast lump sets in train a cavalcade of negative thinking: *'I've got breast cancer! I'll be mutilated. My husband won't love or desire me any more. I'll die! What on earth will happen to the children? I won't see them grow up'*, etc. Figures 3.1 and 3.2 attempt to show the *fear* which suspicion of cancer unleashes. The important question here is *'What does the patient do with his or her fear?'* The logical response to suspicion of serious illness is to see the doctor at the first possible opportunity and some patients do indeed do this. Others are too frightened to have their fears confirmed and decide to wait and see if the symptoms go away. Another important question is *'Whom does the patient tell?'* Some patients will confide at once in their partners but others will keep their fears to themselves in an attempt to spare those they love. Women nursing a dying husband will frequently wait until after he dies before declaring a breast lump, thus reducing their own chance of survival.

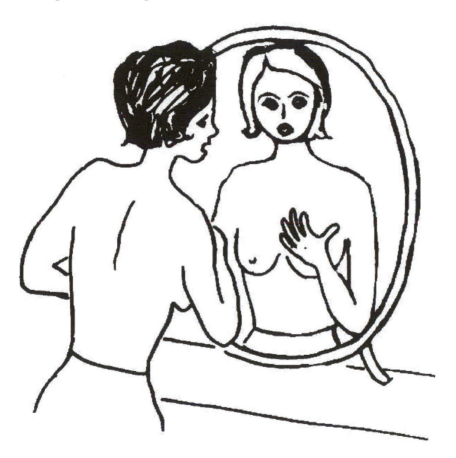

**Figure 3.1**   The first encounter – the suspicion of having cancer. © 2005 Sheila Cassidy.

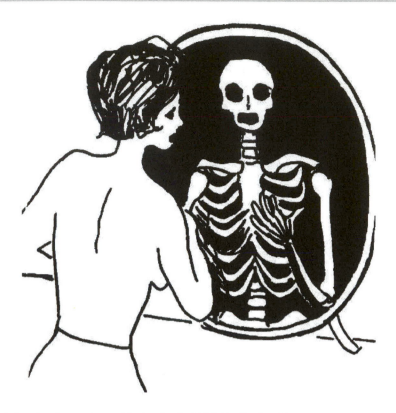

**Figure 3.2**    Confrontation with death. © 2005 Sheila Cassidy.

In the initial assessment of a newly diagnosed cancer patient, it is worth asking the patient about the first moment of suspicion – and how s/he *felt* about it. Not only are the stories illuminating and moving but patient and sympathetic listening is a powerful way to form a *therapeutic alliance*: a good working relationship. The three key questions are:

1  What did you think [when you suspected cancer]?
2  What did you feel [when you suspected cancer]?
3  Whom did you tell [when you suspected cancer]?

Question 3 will let us know if the patient has a *confiding tie*: someone in whom they can confide, such as their mum, sister or a close friend. If a patient has no-one in whom she feels she can confide, then she is psychologically more vulnerable than if she has a close friend whom she can trust. Such lonely patients usually need more professional input than those who are well supported.

## The second encounter

The *second encounter* is with the family doctor when the patient first seeks medical advice about his or her fears (*see* Figure 3.3). Some patients have no problem being 'up-front' about their problems and declare at once, '*I've got a lump in my breast*', or '*I've been passing blood*'. Many people however are shy and embarrassed about their bodily functions and take a while to admit what is their problem. Doctors, of course, pick up this feeling and some may be hesitant in submitting the patient to intimate physical examination. I have vivid and angry memories of a man in his forties whose doctor assumed his rectal bleeding was due to haemorrhoids and did not examine him until his rectal tumour was inoperable. Sometimes, a general practitioner (GP) genuinely believes that a lump is benign but mistakes may cost the patient his or her life.

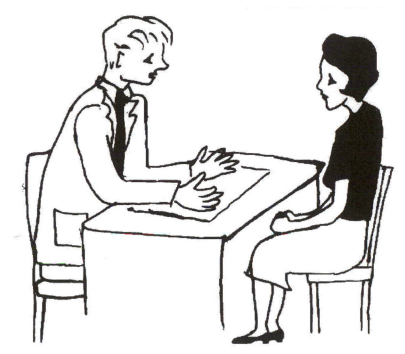

**Figure 3.3**   The second encounter – the GP consultation with the patient. © 2005 Sheila Cassidy.

How the doctor handles the patient who suspects cancer will have a major effect upon that person, for good or for ill. The doctor who makes light of a person's fears effectively shuts him or her up – for who wishes to look foolish in front of someone in authority? The patient needs either firm reassurance or to be told that he or she is right to be concerned. In the latter situation the promise of an urgent hospital appointment will reassure the patient that the necessary steps are being taken.

If the doctor is suspicious that the patient has cancer, s/he should offer to see the patient again with his or her partner so that explanations can be repeated and family support mobilised (*see* Figure 3.4).

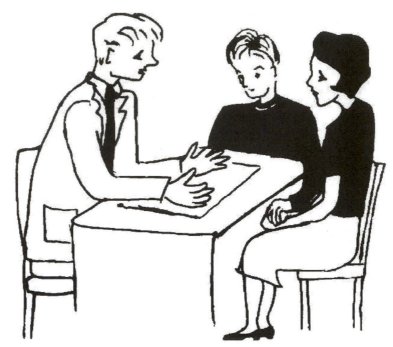

**Figure 3.4**  The second encounter – the GP consultation with the patient and family.
© 2005 Sheila Cassidy.

The *2-week initiative,* in which all patients suspected of having cancer must be seen by a specialist within 14 days, is an important advance, not only in maximising survival but in reducing the time the patient has to worry. However, 2 weeks can feel like a lifetime to an anxious patient, and fear will inevitably disrupt sleep and affect the whole family.

## The third encounter

The *third encounter* is with the specialist and takes place in the often alien hospital environment. The drawing of the consultant (*see* Figure 3.5) dates from the 1980s when nurses wore caps and patients were made to undress and put on hospital dressing gowns before seeing the doctor. This rule of undressing was instituted in good faith to save the doctor's precious time but it was a procedure which stripped a woman of her dignity and increased the power gap between the doctor and the patient. (I still resent putting on the examination gown when I go for my breast cancer check-ups.)

In the oncology department where I helped in the breast cancer clinic for 10 years, the patients undressed only when we needed to examine them. They were in their *own* clothes most of the time.

Like the visits to the GP, this *third encounter* may be helpful or psychologically wounding. If the doctor is kind and friendly, the patient will feel *held* and cherished.

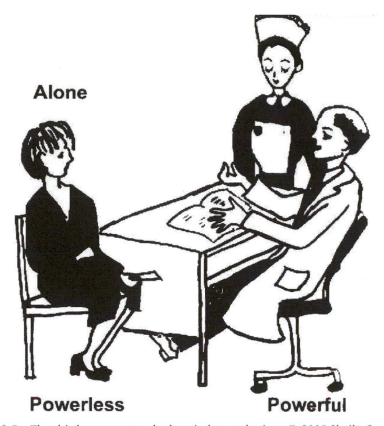

**Alone**

**Powerless**          **Powerful**

**Figure 3.5**   The third encounter – the hospital consultation. © 2005 Sheila Cassidy.

However, if the doctor is cold or pompous and arrogant the patient will be deskilled and humiliated.

I have found the younger generation of consultants to be kinder and more human than many of their forebears and most of the patients I have encountered of recent years speak highly of their specialist. I have, however, vivid memories of the woman who declared: '*They treated me like a lump of meat on a conveyor belt.*' How difficult to balance the human needs of the patient with the ever-increasing demand for speed and efficiency. One such issue is the complaint that, in the hospital outpatient department (OPD), the patient rarely sees the same doctor twice. Having worked for 10 years in the breast cancer clinic where the consultant saw the new patients, and the rest of us (registrar, senior house officer (SHO) and clinical assistants) saw the other patients in order of appointment, I can understand both points of view. As always, there are the demands of training the junior doctors which must be weighed against the psychological needs of the patient. It is in the OPD situation that the staff grade (permanent, non-consultant) doctors can provide continuity for patients undergoing regular hospital follow-up.

It is important to question whether hospital specialists bring far too many patients back for review when they could perhaps be followed up in the community by the GP or specialist nurses. This is particularly relevant in breast cancer patients because metastatic disease often declares itself symptomatically between hospital visits, and early diagnosis, once the disease has spread, is not associated with enhanced survival. (Metastatic is different from primary disease where early diagnosis is of the utmost important to survival.)

## The fourth encounter

The *fourth encounter* is with the knowledge that one has cancer. It may come as the confirmation of suspicion or as a bolt from the blue: a nightmare encounter with the possibility of imminent death. Therefore, the *fourth encounter* is about breaking or confirming bad news. The manner in which this is done will have a profound impact on the patient, which if negative may reverberate around his or her friends and family, increasing the fear of cancer and the distrust of hospitals.

The medical world is full of horror stories of bad news broken insensitively as well as a certain black humour: '*It's the big C: so don't buy any more long-playing gramophone records.*' So why do we find it so difficult to communicate bad news to another? Like most doctors in palliative care, I have done my share of teaching communication skills and there is no doubt that most doctors and nurses are ill at ease with giving patients unpleasant information. There may be a number of reasons for this. The first is that we do not want to hurt people: to cause them mental pain. Second is the fear that people will react violently to such information: that they will 'lose it', faint, become hysterical and that 'we will not be able to cope' with the result. Nurses often talk disparagingly of the way in which doctors break bad news and then leave it to the nurses to 'pick up the pieces'. I would suggest that, providing the doctor does the task sensitively, it is reasonable to ask a nurse to support a distressed patient while s/he processes difficult information. This is partly because doctors in clinics and on ward rounds are under exceptional time pressure and because nurses are often better at the human tasks of comforting than their medical colleagues.

So, how should bad news be broken? This is covered in detail in *Stepping into Palliative Care 2: care and practice*, Chapter 11, but I would suggest there are three key steps:

1 *Find out what the patient knows*, e.g. ask: '*How much do you understand about your illness?*' The answer may be '*It's cancer, isn't it ...*', in which case the reply is gentle confirmation. Alternatively, the patient may say '*Nothing, really ...*', in which case you move to step 2.
2 *Find out what the patient **wants** to know*, e.g. ask: '*Would you like me to explain things to you?*' Here, it is important to pause and listen carefully to the patient's answer. This may be a clear '*Yes, please*', in which case one can proceed with confidence. Alternatively, the patient may be silent or become distressed; in which case I would be very wary and offer a 'get-out clause', such as, '*Would you rather take things one day at a time?*' or '*Would you prefer that I speak to your daughter [husband or someone else]?*' Patients have the right to know what is wrong with them but they also have a right not to have this information forced upon them.
3 *Imparting information.* The third task is the actual imparting of information in a kindly and sensitive manner; as this is done the professional must constantly monitor the patient's understanding, allow them time to process the information and support any emotions which may be triggered.

The following drawings (Figures 3.6 to 3.9) illustrate different situations in which 'bad news' may be given.

- *Figure 3.6* – all good doctors and nurses should know that one should allow patients time to dress before burdening them with important information.
- *Figure 3.7* – here we see the kindly but distant surgeon standing at the foot of the bed, surrounded by his protective entourage of junior doctors and nurses. The ward round is *not* the time to break bad news. This should be done in privacy, without other patients listening behind the curtains, preferably with only one or two observers: the junior doctor because s/he must learn how to do it and the nurse because s/he needs to know what has been said so that s/he can (yes: pick up the pieces!) support the patient when the medics have moved on.
- *Figure 3.8* – this young female doctor is doing her best in a one-to-one interview, and she may be very good – but she will be hampered by lack of life experience and medical knowledge about prognosis. Ideally, a senior doctor or nurse should break bad news.
- *Figure 3.9* – this last drawing of the patient in the bath illustrates the dilemma of the junior nurse who is faced with questions such as '*Have I got cancer, nurse?*' or '*Am I going to die?*' Her answer will depend on the unit where s/he works but such questions will usually need to be passed on to a senior member of staff.

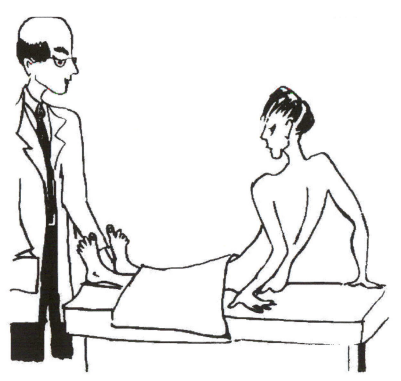

**Figure 3.6**   The fourth encounter – with the knowledge of having cancer. © 2005 Sheila Cassidy.

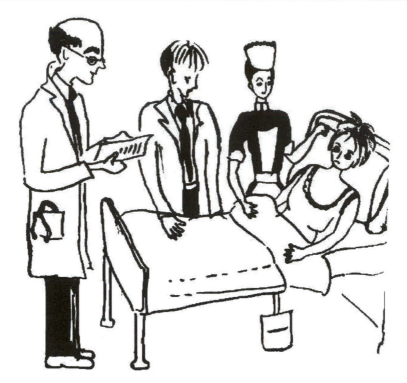

**Figure 3.7**   The ward round. © 2005 Sheila Cassidy.

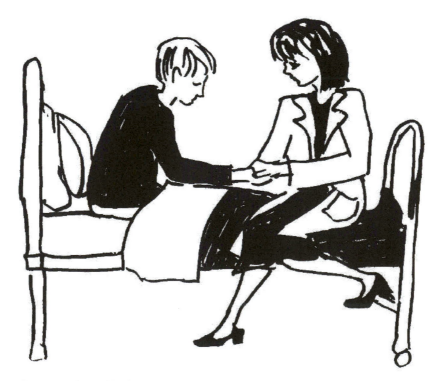

**Figure 3.8**   Breaking bad news. © 2005 Sheila Cassidy.

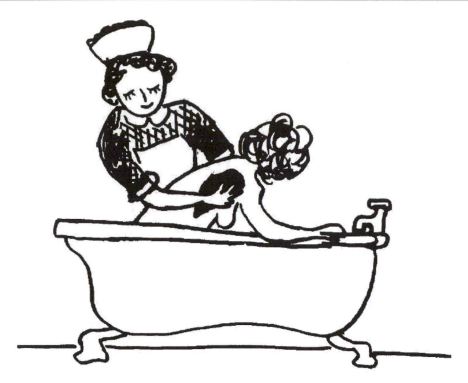

**Figure 3.9**   Talking in privacy. © 2005 Sheila Cassidy.

## The fifth encounter

The *fifth encounter* is with cancer treatment and those who administer it. Treatment may be surgery, radiotherapy, chemotherapy or all three. Each treatment has its own mysteries and side effects and the impact will vary with the experience of the treatment. Lumpectomy for breast cancer should have less impact than mastectomy, although this will depend on how great the mutilation and how the woman feels about it. Bowel surgery requiring a colostomy is likely to have a significant and long-lasting impact because of the disfigurement, inconvenience and embarrassment involved. It is here that the skill of empathy is important: the ability to think, imagine and feel oneself into the patient's world '*as if it were one's own*', so that one's responses may be appropriate and helpful.

Undergoing a course of chemotherapy is famous for being an unpleasant experience. The suffering involved varies from patient to patient, depending on the drugs given and the patient's idiosyncrasy. Some people have a horrible experience with severe vomiting and diarrhoea while others on the same regime can keep working with only brief periods off sick. Having said that, the majority of young women with primary breast cancer who attended the support group (which I ran over a period of 7 years) were off work for the best part of a year: having surgery, recovering from surgery, undergoing 6 months of chemotherapy and then, after a month, 6 weeks of radiotherapy.

The treatment experience is not all bad and many patients find the love and care given by friends, family and professionals to be truly heart warming and life giving.

## When the treatment is over

When treatment is safely over, convalescence begins and all concerned should be duly thankful. The professionals move on to care for someone else, but ... *what about the patient and family?*

In my experience, after the initial days of recovery, convalescence feels unbearably slow. *There seems an enormous gulf between being 'better' by medical standards and feeling normal by the patients' standards.* Although grateful that all has gone well, patients lack their normal energy and joy in living. This is not helped by the attitude of their nearest and dearest who either *wrap them in cotton wool,* or expect them to be back to normal long before that is possible.

Apart from these very human misunderstandings, there is always the ongoing fear of recurrence of the original cancer. Every ache and pain, every lump and bump is cancer until proved otherwise – a state of mind which can be quite irritating to both family and professionals. It is here that patience and empathy from the professional is important if the patient is not to feel neurotic and foolish.

Because of this natural fear of recurrence, each outpatient check-up, especially the early ones, can be enormously stressful. It is always a delight to me as a doctor to be able to reassure patients that all is well and tell them they need not come again for 6 months or a year (*see* Figure 3.10).

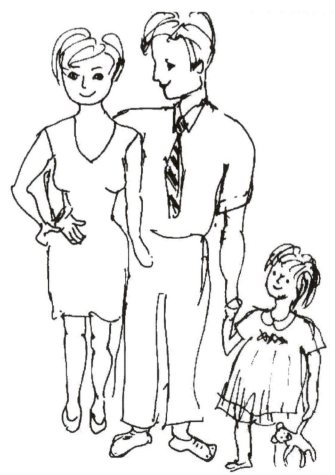

**Figure 3.10**   Many patients are cured. © 2005 Sheila Cassidy.

Inevitably, in some patients, disease *does* return and, for many, this is the beginning of their *terminal* illness, their *journey* towards death. With luck and good management, palliative treatment may last for several years and the truly *terminal* illness kept at bay. Much of the work of the clinic in which I worked was palliative and the consultant was skilled at maintaining quality of life by the use of small doses of less toxic chemotherapy. In modern oncology centres, the emphasis is on quality of life rather than length of days and patients are managed with sensitivity and openness.

## The sixth encounter

The *sixth encounter* (*see* Figure 3.11) is with the knowledge that the disease is no longer curable. As a cancer patient myself, with a high statistical chance of survival, I find it surprisingly difficult to put myself in the shoes of those whose hopes are suddenly dashed. When I began working in oncology 25 years ago, doctors thought it wrong to take hope away so they lied and lied about their ability to cure people and thus saved themselves the pain of breaking bad news. This deception works fine for a while as patients respond to treatment but, as relapse is followed by relapse, most people realise that they are losing the battle. How then must they feel when the specialist goes on promising cure while they themselves know that they are losing ground daily? The answer is that such people feel unbearably lonely and are confused and are prevented from talking to those they love about their most urgent problem: the fact that they are going to die.

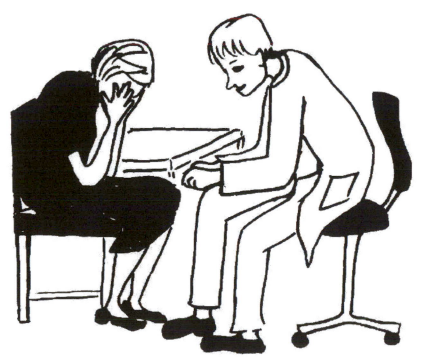

**Figure 3.11**   The sixth encounter – breaking bad news that disease has recurred. © 2005 Sheila Cassidy.

When I began working as an SHO on the oncology wards in 1980, I used to do an evening ward round and spend time, especially, with the patients in the side wards, many of whom were dying. As we sat together, the patients would often find the courage to ask that most difficult of questions: '*Am I going to die, doctor?*' In that almost confessional atmosphere, I found it impossible to lie so I learnt to speak the truth, however painful. The gratitude of these men and women was enormous: they had been isolated for months by *the conspiracy of silence* – the decision of their families and doctors to 'protect' them by keeping the truth from them. This was, for me, the beginning of true palliative care in which pretence is dropped and the patient *accompanied* rather than clinically observed.

After 11 years as medical director of Plymouth's St Luke's Hospice, I returned to work in oncology where I provided a one-woman palliative care service to the rest of the hospital. The initial vision was that I should teach the junior doctors how to manage the terminally ill but the reality was that they were too busy to spend the time needed. What the nurses wanted from me was to tell their patients the truth about their situation: usually that there was no further curative treatment on offer. (All this was around 15 years ago and, hopefully, such situations are managed better now.)

To go in 'cold' and tell a stranger that s/he is going to dies seems barbaric, so I would spend as much time as was needed to get to know the patient before broaching the issue of the future. In particular, I found out about their family, who was 'there' with them and who depended on them. In the space of 40 minutes or so, I was able to establish a good rapport with the patient so that when the time came to discuss the future they felt they could trust me. Such work was time consuming and emotionally draining but infinitely worthwhile because knowing the truth nearly always brought peace to the patient and family. Commonly, the patient would ask to go home that day so that s/he could spend precious time in their own space with those they loved.

## Living with a terminal illness

I am referring now to the months and weeks between the moments of realisation that death is inevitable and the actual moment of death. Different people, depending on the nature of their illness and the care available, will spend this period in different places. A patient with motor neurone disease may spend many months in a hospice or nursing home as may patients with multiple bone deposits who require round-the-clock nursing. However, the majority of cancer patients spend most of their time at home with occasional visits to the hospice or the oncology clinic (*see* Figure 3.12). The life of the latter group of patients has been transformed by the advent of the 'Macmillan nurse,' the community clinical nurse specialising in psychological and symptom management of terminally ill patients in their own homes. When pain and other unpleasant symptoms are well managed, even gravely ill patients can enjoy a reasonable quality of life: indeed, some may continue working until shortly before they die.

When St Luke's in Plymouth opened its first seven beds in 1982, we thought that those patients we admitted would stay with us until they died. We had no idea that within 10 years we would be running a highly specialised, 20-bedded unit for the management of symptoms in the terminally ill. Nor would we have believed that

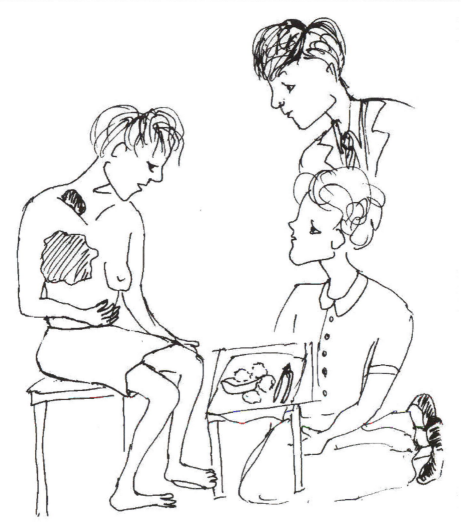

**Figure 3.12**  Palliative care team – symptom control and psychological support. © 2005 Sheila Cassidy.

most patients would stay no longer than 2 weeks and would return home or go to a nursing home.

Although the development of professional expertise in pain and other symptom management has greatly improved the care of the terminally ill, the demand for hospice beds has increased way beyond that which could have been predicted. This means that the vision of hospice as a place for long-term care of the terminally ill is no longer viable, except in a few cases requiring specialised nursing. Those patients who cannot be cared for at home will end their days not in the hospice but in a nursing home.

In theory, care in the nursing home should be as good as in the hospice but financial constraints imposed by running a business make this difficult to achieve. In Plymouth, where I have worked for the past 25 years, we have for several years had an active programme of education in palliative care for nursing home staff. This year an experienced Macmillan nurse has been appointed as a resource to local nursing homes so we are hopeful that this will increase the confidence and expertise of this group of carers.

## The seventh – final – encounter

The *seventh* and *final encounter* (*see* Figure 3.13) is with death: the end of life – or perhaps the beginning, depending on what you believe.

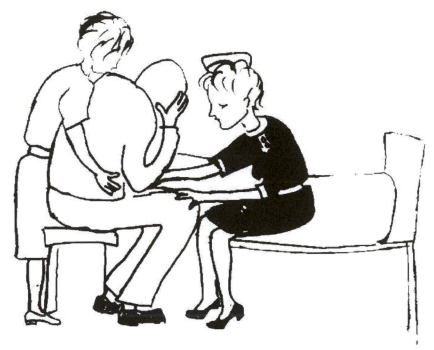

**Figure 3.13**   The seventh encounter – the moment of death. © 2005 Sheila Cassidy.

Once the patient has been made as comfortable as possible, our concerns must be to support the family. We need to know if they wish to accompany the dying person in his or her last hours, and if they do, we must keep an unobtrusive but watchful eye on them, providing refreshment and comfort as required. In a hospice, this care is taken for granted, but in the general hospital, things may be different. I have heard relatives speak of sitting with their dying relative throughout the night without being offered as much as a cup of tea. I know it is asking a lot of two young night nurses in charge of a busy ward to provide tea and sympathy but such courtesies are the least we can offer at such a pivotal time in people's lives. People remember the death of their loved ones in detail and grieving is inevitably complicated by anger and bitterness if care is perceived as having been inadequate. It is worth remembering that relatives frequently suffer post-traumatic stress syndrome with intrusive flashbacks of their loved ones' features in their dying moments. Therefore, *good care of the dying includes good care of the living who love them* (*see* Figure 3.14).

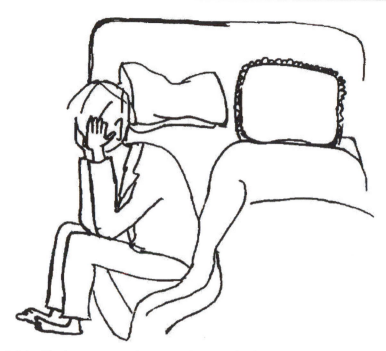

**Figure 3.14**    The bereavement journey. © 2005 Sheila Cassidy.

## Conclusion

I hope that in *travelling* on this *cancer journey* you have developed some insight into how it feels to be a cancer patient. Psychotherapist Carl Rogers in his book *On Becoming a Person* describes the *core conditions* for a good therapeutic relationship as:

- transparency
- empathy
- unconditional positive regard.

*Transparency* asks that we drop our professional façade and be 'alongside' the patient as another human being.

*Empathy*, which I see as the key to all good caring, demands that we develop the ability to '*enter into the other's world as if it were one's own, without losing the "as if" quality*'. It is only by walking in our patients' shoes that we can know what they need and how we should respond. The phase '*without losing the "as if" quality*' means that we always retain the knowledge that the person we are treating is not a relative or a close friend: if we do that, our work may drain but will not overwhelm us.

The last of the core conditions is *unconditional positive regard*, and asks that we continue to accept and value our patients despite their many human frailties.

My last word, as an old hand in palliative care, is that *you look after yourself*, because if you don't, who will look after the patient? Take all your leave and time off, and have as much fun as you can, because then you will bring light and laughter to the frightened and the grieving.

## To learn more

- Cassidy SA. *Sharing the Darkness: the spirituality of caring*. London: Darton Longman and Todd; 1988.
- Cassidy SA. *Light from the Dark Valley*. London: Darton Longman and Todd; 1994.
- Cassidy SA. *The Loneliest Journey*. London: Darton Longman and Todd; 1995.
- Rogers C. *On Becoming a Person: a therapist's view of psychotherapy*. Boston: Houghton Mifflin; 1995.
- Wright S, Sayre-Adams J. *Sacred Space – right relationship and spirituality in health care*. Churchill Livingstone, London; 2000.

## Complementary chapters

*See also Stepping into Palliative Care 1: relationships and responses*

- Chapter 5: The psychological impact of serious illness
- Chapter 6: Hope and coping strategies
- Chapter 7: The therapeutic relationship
- Chapter 9: Integrated care pathways

*See also Stepping into Palliative Care 2: care and practice*

- Chapter 1: Assessment in palliative care
- Chapter 9: The last few days of life
- Chapter 11: Breaking bad news
- Chapter 13: Spirituality and palliative care
- Chapter 16: The special needs of the neurological patient

# Chapter 4

# The experience of illness

*Oliver Slevin*

## Preamble

Shortly after I had commenced working on this chapter, my father died. At one point during a period of many days of breath-gasping and tortuous decline, there was one moment when he stared at me with what seemed to be desperate and desolate realisation. It was as if, in my returning gaze, I had in that instant looked into the very soul of someone in torment and was devoid of any meaningful response either to him or myself. I was reminded of Henri Nouwen's[1] account of his own mother's similarly painful death: *'an experience that to be described would require words that have not yet been found'*.

## Introduction

In this chapter we are primarily concerned with the experience of illness – that is, how we become conscious of a phenomenon (illness), and then how we make sense of this. This emphasises three conditions: first, experience is empirical, in so far as it relates to some object or occurrence that we become aware of; second, it is something that is personal, or contained within the self – only the individual truly knows what s/he experiences; third, we are drawn to attempt to make sense of what we experience, to discern meaning.

It is also important, before we even proceed to what we mean by illness – and how it relates to other phenomena such as health, disease and wellbeing – to consider the parameters of our discussion within the chapter. In addressing illness as an experience, we might consider the following:

- *Who* it is that is experiencing the phenomenon. There is of course the person who is personally experiencing illness – the person suffering or afflicted. But there are also others who experience this phenomenon, albeit indirectly, as the close relatives, partners or friends of the individual, or as professionals responding to the person's need.
- *What* is being experienced. Here also the primary person affected is the individual who is ill, and the concern is to establish exactly what that individual is experiencing. But others – for example, a spouse or partner – also experience something when a loved one becomes distressed, incapacitated, perhaps even commences the journey toward death.
- *How* the experience is responded to. This, as we shall see, relates to our more direct responses to the symptoms that occur (pain, breathlessness, nausea, etc.), perhaps by seeking relief or cure. It also relates to the way in which we attempt to

make sense of, or attribute meaning to, what is happening to us. These two are not of course mutually exclusive.

- *When* and *where* the illness experience occurs. This identifies how the variables of time and space impact upon the experience. The issue here is predominantly one of culture.[2] Within modern Western societies it is most likely that the individual will see his/her illness experience in terms of a scientific biomedical model. It is assumed that some disease (an infection, or cancer, or metabolic imbalance) is the cause of the onset of *unwellness*. However, at different times or in different places, other explanations may prevail – a deity has punished the person for wrongdoing, or a witch has cast a spell. Indeed, even in our own Western culture, those of a more extreme fundamentalist orientation may see some sufferers as wicked; and conditions such as AIDS (acquired immune deficiency syndrome) as God's retribution for wrongdoing.[3,4]

The space available in this brief chapter does not permit a detailed consideration of all these matters. Instead, attention is given to the first three of the above – the matters of who, what and how; and, in respect of the first of these, we will concern ourselves primarily with the individual experiencing illness, whom we term *the sufferer* or *the one afflicted*. We also assume that the person so identified is progressing through a disease that is severe and indeed life-threatening, or who is even in the terminal stages of such a disease.

## On illness and disease

It is sometimes claimed that the issue concerning the medical profession, and indeed other healthcare professions, is that of *disease* – that is, pathological changes within the body (or indeed mind). Conversely, what the afflicted person is experiencing, including those experiences that are termed *symptoms*, is that phenomenon we term *illness*. The person who is ill is said to experience a bad feeling. Indeed, the original old European root of the word ill is 'feeling bad'. This is at first a little confusing. After all, the word 'disease' is itself indicative of a lack of ease, a term that in old French denoted pleasure or comfort. However, in modern usage, 'disease' is a term almost always reserved for the pathological condition of body or mind that causes such negative feeling or lack of ease.

It might thus be argued that there is a difference between disease and illness, particularly if we accept that the former is a disordered condition of mind or body while the latter is the experience that this usually elicits in the sufferer. Disease, to a large extent, is something that is circumscribed. We might see it in terms of a malfunctioning (diseased) heart or liver, or in terms of a virus infection of our respiratory tract. However, the experience of illness resides in the person, or the self, not in an individual body organ. Illness is '*what the patient feels when he goes to the doctor*' while disease is '*what the patient has on the way home from the doctor's office*'.[5]

A further consideration is that how we experience illness is itself a complex phenomenon. We might argue, and indeed this is generally the case, that the illness experience is negative. As we note above, the origins of the word *ill* is associated with 'badness' in the sense of 'feeling bad'. However, illness *may* involve positive experiences. We are aware that some mental illnesses are characterised by what are adjudged abnormally high levels of elation or ecstasy. Indeed, conditions such as anorexia nervosa, while commonly associated with extreme distress and depression, may in some instances involve an element of pleasure in self-denial and self-harm. The idea of a *sick role*[6] may allow one to relinquish all other roles and adopt a passive dependent role. This incorporates within it an unburdening comfort, but at the same time may have implications for the extent to which the individual confronts their illness. Despite such risks, resistance to adopting a dependent and compliant role is often viewed negatively and discouraged by carers.[7]

Importantly, the experience of illness at the level of 'self' or 'being' might also have certain positive attributes. As we are confronted with the reality of our own mortality, and as we seek meaning to our lives, we may achieve high levels of enlightenment and spiritual wellbeing. Such heightened enlivenment may have been lost to us in a previously hectic and unrewarding lifestyle, more characterised by a sense of alienation than fulfilment. The illness experience may distress us and indeed may herald our early demise, but at the same time may be life-enhancing and transformational.

It is important that in all of this we do not lapse into some dualistic separation of the notions of disease and illness as opposing positions, particularly where postmodern arguments present the concept of disease as primarily a negative and depersonalising device. We know that in some instances the approach to disease in the much-maligned 'medical model' can be a mechanical, objectified and impersonal undertaking that literally excludes the sufferer as person. We know also that the medicalisation of modern society carries the risk of a medical explanation being used for almost any deviation from the norm, sometimes even to the extent of medicine becoming an instrument of social control.[8–10] But let us be quite clear on this point at least: there is no illness, and no illness experience in the first place, if there is not an underlying disease at its root. They are, in effect, two sides of the same coin. Furthermore, a conception of disease that excludes from its consideration what the sufferer is experiencing and feeling as a person is by definition incomplete.

---

**Reflective exercise 4.1: Illness in context**
**Time: 30 minutes**

1  Do a brief literature search of the terms illness, disease, sickness, health and wellbeing.
2  Reflect on differences and similarities in the terms.
3  Then re-read the latter section of the chapter in a more critical fashion, considering additional points you feel might be made.

---

## The journey into experience

From this point, we can consider the journey into and through illness further. Those of us who are now ill, and perhaps even seriously ill, are, so to speak, en route. You may recognise the journey plotted below. Perhaps you will be able to say '*Ah yes, that is what it is like!*' or alternatively '*No, you are not even beginning to see, you would've had to have been there!*' We can only say this: the narrative presented here is the author's construction. Those who have not yet been seriously ill can only glimpse it through the stories of others, and as Arthur Frank[11] demonstrated, for each of these others their story is or was to some extent unique.

Space does not allow us to dwell on context and cultural issues, nor indeed the experience of others in relationships with the ill person. Instead, we make assumptions that the context is the experiencing of serious illness within our Western modern society. In this context we are concerned with the ill person, what he or she may be experiencing, and how he or she responds to such experiences. As presented here, there *is* a sense in which there is a journey that indeed has its stages from beginning to end. But at the same time, the journey is convoluted, with its stages running into and around each other, and with much movement forward and backwards. This journey does indeed begin with an awareness that is at its beginning the mere sensing that all is not well. But awareness continues with the ill person throughout the journey, as they become aware of the seriousness of their plight, and later of a turning point towards recovery or alternatively a decline towards death. Nevertheless, while we recognise that this journey may be experienced as entering a world of chaos rather than a neatly plotted trip, it serves our purpose to address the elements making up the experience of illness in a more orderly fashion.

## Awareness

There is something in the nature of a *consciousness* here, an intentional focus upon something that is different, a change that has taken place. All is not well, something is happening. To the clinician, the situation may be viewed as the emergence or appearance of symptoms. But to the individual, this awareness is of a deeply personal nature. Sometimes the thing now noticed, the change happening, has a cultural significance: it is a *known* and dreaded phenomenon. The individual may be proceeding as normal, involved in the everyday. Then perhaps, while showering, she notices a lump in her breast. To women in our Western society, this has definite connotations, as the possibility of a breast cancer burgeons in upon the individual's consciousness. The range of emotions immediately experienced and the speed of their passage may be shattering in their immediacy: sudden anxiety, a dread of the implications, a panic setting in. The individual is struck by a sense of disbelief and denial. But there it is: '*I have checked again; it is definitely a lump. Oh my God, this can't be happening to me. Why me? What will I do?*'

Of course, it does not always happen like this. For everyone it is different. There may be a gradual consciousness of tiredness and lack of energy. Even previously easy tasks like climbing the staircase now cause breathlessness. There is a dry hacking cough that seems not to be going away. But still, and for a time, the person pushes these experiences off, rationalises them in terms of a virus infection or overwork. However, as time passes, and as the problems do not go away but in fact increase in severity, there is this eventually unavoidable awareness – that all is not well, that in fact something is seriously wrong.

## Being and non-being

What is happening can perhaps best be understood in terms of how each of us experiences how we are in the world. The German philosopher Martin Heidegger[12] referred to this as '*being-in-the-world*'. The German term he used for this existent person or entity, or indeed state of being, was *Dasein*. This translates as *'there-being'*, being there or existing as a self or entity. For Heidegger, there were two ways of being – *authentic* and *inauthentic*. It is important that negative attributes are not attached to what Heidegger termed the *'inauthentic'*. He was not concerned with that sense in which inauthenticity suggests falsehood or untrustworthiness, but with something like avoiding confronting our own realities. For him, this was the normal way of being in day-to-day living. In effect each of us find a security in the social world we inhabit: it has a structure and recognised processes; within it we find relationships in work, family and friendship; there is a sense of stability and constancy, an almost illusory experiencing of order in our world and our place within it; it is something that is permanent and has a sense of infinity about it. This social web, to which we relate and of which we are a part, Heidegger described as *das Man* (meaning *'the Other'*). This is explained by seeing the individual as the One-Self, in relation to 'they' or the 'other', with which the One-Self is at one. Thus, we work 'as one does', we establish relationships 'as one does', etc., in line with the culture and social context.

The converse of this, *authentic* being, has no 'One-Self', but rather an 'I-Self'. The individual here experiences being 'thrown-into-the-world' as a separate being who has, in the final analysis, only the self and the self's resources to call upon. This awareness by the individual as a being who exists alone and apart from others carries with it an acute awareness not only of the fact that as a person 'I exist', but also that as a person at some time 'I will cease to exist'. Existence or *being* thus carries with it the unavoidable awareness of the prospect of *nothingness*. This is experienced as a sense of anxiety that relates to our separateness and isolation from all others and, in the final analysis, our death or non-being.

Unsurprisingly, all of us seek the security of the inauthentic way of being. Heidegger was himself at pains to suggest that no one could tolerate living within the angst of constant authentic being. According to Young,[13] inauthentic being:

> is tranquilizing since ... one is 'disburdened' of a disturbing weight which anyone who lives as an 'I-Self,' as an individual, must bear. This weight, says Heidegger, is death: the inexorable mortality of each individual. In its most fundamental description, therefore, inauthentic life is a flight from death.[13]

Of course, it is impossible to avoid the authentic way of being. From time to time we are thrust into an awareness of our own mortality, and increasingly so as we get older. Most frequently these are fleeting moments from which we escape by a return to the routine and 'normality' of everyday inauthentic living. But for the person who is experiencing a serious and perhaps terminal illness, this enhanced sense of existing as a mortal being becomes not only pronounced but also unavoidable as a constant reminder. The individual experiences the sensations of pain and perhaps the increasing severity of this. Furthermore, the individual has been made aware, at some stage in the diagnostic process, that this can be attributed to a disease that may also have been defined as not only fatal but terminal. As such awareness is repeatedly called to consciousness, a confrontation with authentic being, each return to the inauthentic life of the everyday is accompanied by an ever-increasing awareness of its illusory and transitory nature. In effect, the illusion, so to speak, sustains us less and less, and we are constantly called by this critical realisation to the authentic state. In a sense, the sufferer is moving from a position of *awareness* to one of *realisation* and even *acceptance*.

---

**Reflective exercise 4.2: Loneliness**
**Time: 30 minutes**

1 Find yourself a quiet space and reflect on what it means to be really lonely.
2 Try to imagine what differences there may be between this and other experiences such as solitude or togetherness.
3 Imagine or relive an occasion when you experienced loneliness and the feelings you recall experiencing.

---

## Separation: confronting mortality alone

To the ill person, there is the often a realisation that there has been a *status passage*, that s/he is now different and apart. To others also (relatives, friends, professionals), there is a sense in which there is this ill person who is now different and apart from us. At this point a barrier snaps into place. To the ill person on one side, s/he may experience a separation from all others and the sense of dissociation, loneliness and perhaps even desolation that can accompany this. To those on the other side the ill person becomes a focus of attention in a new way. There is of course a cognitive awareness of the change in the 'ill' other, and this may be accompanied by something we might term concern or compassion. But this is often accompanied by a sense of awe. What is happening to the ill person is in an experiential sense beyond our ken; we may gaze into this world of pain and suffering but we are not really a part of it.

All of us can appreciate, at a cognitive level, what is happening when someone falls under a bus. At a more emotive level, we can relate to the trauma that ensues, and we may even empathise through association with some injury we have sustained in the past. But only the person under the bus feels, actually feels, the crunch of bones, something ripping within the body, the sudden horror of things coming apart, the drift into unconsciousness. So too with the illness of others as we – the 'non-ill' – countenance it. It is the other that is on the other side of the barrier, the other that is 'under the bus'. The person experiencing illness is therefore, as an authentic being, alone on his or her journey. That person must confront his or her own existence and his or her own prospective non-existence. That is not to say that others cannot reach a hand across the divide, cannot experience at least some awareness of the plight of the sufferer, cannot say that to as great an extent as possible they will be there – in their place by the sufferer's side – as the sufferer confronts his or her destiny. Nevertheless the separation of the sick from the well, and the eventual removal to the sick room or place of dying, may have a purpose of providing peace and solitude, but can in reality increase the sense of loneliness and isolation.[14]

## The lived experience of suffering

Thus we find this person: confronted by an illness, plucked from his or her 'inauthentic' existence, and set apart as a self that must endure. We have already acknowledged that to be ill is to 'feel bad'. Indeed, we have already alluded to this person as the sufferer. But what does it mean to suffer? What is it that is being suffered? To suffer is to endure. That is in fact the basis of the word's Latin roots.

There is the physical sense of enduring or experiencing pain but also the emotional sense of experiencing sadness and distress.[15] Both of these can be of almost unbearable proportions. We may all have experienced the raging pain of a tooth-ache or the excruciating pain of a headache. But the intractable pain that may be experienced in a terminal illness may be such that it defines the very totality of one's tortured consciousness from moment to moment. In addition, the sense of sadness and loss experienced by the awareness of an illness from which – it may be perceived – there is no recovery and no future also carries its own distress that can be defined as suffering.

There are still other aspects of suffering that might be seen as an assault on the embodied self. In a modern world health and wellbeing, and the body beautiful, are almost single-minded aspirations. There is a stigma in illness; it bears a mark that sets the ill person at once apart and not only different but flawed. The scarred face, the mutilated body following breast surgery, or the horror of the attached colostomy bag, all become sources of profound shame. The individual feels not only embarrassed but also dishonoured and wishes only to hide his or her unsightliness or uncleanness from others. This may even be accompanied by feelings of guilt, as with the habitual smoker or person who has contracted AIDS. It is not only shameful that one is ill, but also doubly shameful because it is one's fault.[16,17] Such attribution of cause to agency on the part of the sufferer is not only confined to the latter examples, but may torture a person with any serious disease: was it something I have done? Is this God's retribution for wrongful living?

The person so afflicted may already be moving into the passive sick role referred to earlier. Now, not only grasped in authentic dread and existential loneliness, the person perhaps feels not only the pain of physical suffering and the emotions of sadness or anxiety, but also the shame of illness and the guilt of its association. Like Chiron, the original wounded healer of Greek mythology, the person withdraws to his own cave of suffering. In this state, there may be a wavering between on the one hand hope and agency, where (as did Chiron, eventually) the individual seeks a way out of this predicament, and on the other hand hopelessness and loss of agency, where there seems no way forward other than to endure as best one can. What is happening here? The person is above all enduring. But this enduring can be in silence and hidden from the world, or in a crying out. And it can be avoided through denial, or confronted (as in the case of Chiron) in a search for meaning and even as a quest for hope.[18]

---

Reflective exercise 4.3: The wounded healer
Time: 20 minutes

It is argued in one of the texts cited in this chapter (*see* Henri Nouwen's text, *The Wounded Healer*[19]) that it is only through suffering ourselves that we can relate with true compassion to the suffering of others. In the Chiron myth it was his quest for liberation from his own suffering that made him so helpful to others.

1 Look up the Chiron myth.
2 Do a brief review of literature on the 'wounded healer' theme.

3 Reflect upon how your experience of life and suffering may make you more sensitive and responsive to the suffering of others:
a When reflecting upon sensitivity, consider your capacity for *empathy*.
b When reflecting upon responsiveness, consider your capacity for *compassion* – and how you really attend to others, not only to their communications but also to their silences.

## Avoiding reality and seeking meaning

As the individual proceeds through an illness there may be a great need to understand, to discern some sense of meaning in respect of what is happening. However, this is not always the case. Here again authentic and inauthentic being becomes an issue. Confronted by the painful experience of illness, the knowledge of a serious and perhaps terminal disease, and the sense of loneliness and desolation all of this engenders, the sufferer may try to escape into the inauthentic world. There may be an attempt to become immersed in and seek comfort from the routine and order of the everyday. The individual may continue, for as long as possible, to work and engage in social activities and relationships. It is important to note again that this is not some abnormal or weak response. As we noted earlier, even Heidegger recognised that this is how we must survive, for it is impossible to live always in the angst of authentic being.

Even the world of healthcare, into which the sufferer is eventually thrust, seems to collude in the construction of the illusion. This is a world of diagnostic tests, problem-oriented discussions among clinicians and between them and the sufferer, the routines of outpatient appointments and inpatient trajectories. All of these combine to reconstruct the illness journey as an objectified disease journey. This also serves to maintain the inauthentic, to keep the authentic at bay, from both sufferer and carers. And it must be recognised that this too has its useful purpose – it provides a space within which the sufferer and those who help can address in reasoned and scientific ways how the course of a disease might be attenuated or indeed reversed.

Notwithstanding such 'normal' responses, it is also possible that the sufferer goes through phases that may be described as less healthy responses: anger and resentment; attempts to dissociate emotions from clear causes for concern; denial or refusal to acknowledge the worsening situation; or, despair, depression and thoughts of the ultimate escape through self-destruction. It is important that such responses are not condemned out of hand as being inappropriate. Within particular contexts, and for particular individuals, this may be the only way of coping at a particular time. Michael Kearney[20] describes how some terminally ill individuals do seek to understand and come to grips with the situation, while others may continue, perhaps for the duration of the illness, to adopt a constant position of denial.

For the sufferer, and indeed those close to him or her, it is at this point usually insufficient to take what has come to pass as merely some sort of existential given: I was well and am now ill; I was alive and am now dying. It is a characteristic of humans, as opposed to other animals, that we *do* have concept of illness, recovery, death and dying, and that we seek something that we might term *meaning* in this respect. Unfortunately, like so many of the terms in this chapter, meaning may have different definitions. For our purpose, it is useful to see the term as referring to signifiers or signs (pieces of information) that indicate something to be understood. Furthermore, it is suggested that in crude terms this can be viewed at both a surface or superficial level, and a fundamental or deep level. At a surface level we may seek, in a largely cognitive sense, an understanding of the disease that underlies our illness: what has caused it, its nature and severity, how the treatment works, and – importantly – the anticipated effectiveness of such interventions. But meaning in a deeper sense is rather different. We seek a meaningful life and thus also a meaningfulness to the end of life. We dread a meaningless or worthless life and a death that – by virtue of untimeliness or accident – also appears to lack meaning. For some, this seeking after meaning may be described as a spiritual phenomenon, while others may describe it as a journey of self-discovery.[21]

The recognition of a deeper 'inner self' is widely recognised in Western psychology. The psychotherapist James Hillman[22] speaks of an inner being that is enlivening, an energy or soul that is sustaining yet requires sustenance. In the East, Chan Buddhism recognises four ways we know that are progressively deeper: information acquisition; seeking and achieving truth; intersubjective knowledge in our relations with others; and, at the deepest level, self-knowledge that at one level may be reflected upon but at a more fundamental level is a tacit knowing of oneself in the world.[23] These levels are not mutually exclusive but nevertheless acknowledge an inner self. In a sense, at the surface level the concern is with what is happening to one and why, while at the deep level the concern is with such matters as what it means to live, what it means to die, what happens when one dies.

---

**Reflective exercise 4.4: A self within?**
**Time: 30 minutes**

1  Contemplate who you really are. Do you subscribe to the idea that there is an inner you, and do you see this as a soul, or psyche, or inner self?
2  While doing this, relax as much as possible. Try to let material thoughts and awareness of your environment drift away. What is left? Is this that remains simply sensations you are aware of, or do you experience a sense of being that seems to transcend such stimuli?

---

## Living life as it is given, facing illness and death as it approaches

How each individual seeks meaning in such circumstances is itself a highly individual experience. It is important to recognise that this can relate to meaning in different contexts: meaning the person attributes to their past life; meaning they attribute to the life that is now being lived as an ill and perhaps terminally ill person; and meaning in terms of death as an approaching human phenomenon.

### Appraising the past

In such circumstances, an individual may be led to reflect upon their past life. Did one lead a good life? Has one made a valuable contribution to the lives of others? Are there lost chances or unfinished business that are now to be lost forever? It has been suggested that the suffering of someone already in pain and distress who is perhaps also faced with the prospect of dying becomes even more distressing if they feel their whole life has been a failure, or if they feel intense remorse about unresolved matters. Indeed, Michael Kearney[20] describes how such agitation and torment may even lead to poor responsiveness to analgesia in palliative care, while conversely coming to terms with one's past and present predicament may result in reductions in the need for analgesic therapy.

## Living now

How a person lives in the shadow of a serious disease will vary widely. This is largely a function of the person's state of mind and the extent to which they have come to terms with the situation (or indeed seek shelter in denial). It is also conditional on the nature of the disease and its progression. Clearly, where a person is in the terminal stages of an illness, driven with pain or needing support with breathing, the horizons may be limited to the immediate environment of the sick bed. But with modern-day advances, one is more often provided not only with the protective cloak of palliative care, but also the space this affords to reflect upon how one will live.

In such circumstances, one person may determine to maintain a normal lifestyle to as great an extent as is possible, perhaps even taking time to achieve something not previously accomplished. Another may seek solace in a spiritual peace made possible by their religious or humanistic beliefs, and prayer or immersion in the presence of loved ones may be their way. Yet another may live in constant angst, torment and fear, wishing only for the oblivion afforded by sleep and analgesia. Someone who has no loved ones or friends, who feels they have largely led a valueless life, may feel extremely distressed at the prospect of the remaining time left. This is perhaps the most dreaded prospect, that of ending one's days alone and uncared for, with no future and perhaps also a past that can only torment one in the final days and hours. It has even been suggested that someone who has lost all sense of meaning in life may expire, when a recovery would otherwise be reasonable to expect.[19,24] Conversely, a young terminally ill mother, concerned about the welfare of her children, may astonish the medical experts by her determination to survive for them as long as possible. The most experienced and eminent of our clinicians recognise something they may term the loss of a will to live, and also the opposite determination to survive. There indeed seems to be some life-force within each of us that must itself be kindled by some sense of meaning or purpose for survival.

## Facing the end

It is important to recognise that death as an experience is an unknown. Yet we do know some things about it. Death is *final*: even for those who have faith in an afterlife there is a recognition that this life will end. Death is a *constant* and *equitable presence*: each of us potentially may or may not have been born successfully, but once born each and all of us *will* die. Death and dying is *uncertain*: leaving aside accounts of near-death experiences, none of us really know the experience of dying; and, whether we believe in nihilistic nothingness or a hereafter, none of us in reality know what, if anything, will occur or remain, or for how long – in terms of a consciousness, or soul, or self, or spirit – when that phenomenon we define as death occurs.

The end can therefore mean different things to different people. Those with belief in God and a strong faith in a hereafter may believe that they confront not a final end at all but a passage into another mode of existence. Others who hold no such belief may take comfort instead in more humanistic beliefs – that they have made a difference to others and that the good they have done in this world, and the tenderness felt for them and by them, will live on. Yet others may see no comfort in such sources of hope or sustenance; to them death may be simply the dismal end to what (as suggested earlier) has become viewed as a dismal existence and worthless life.

We may not wish to leave the matter here. There is tidiness to the workings of the human mind that seeks completion, a final position that is palatable. At all costs we seek something of at least a glimmer of hope, to find at least some small element of silver lining to the cloud. Sometimes we *do* find this. There *are* instances of what Elisabeth Kubler-Ross[25] describes as 'a peaceful death', and we hope this is more often the case. But those in the death business know that this is not always so. Bert Keizer[26] ends his uncompromising *Dancing with Mister D* with the quotation: '*Maybe he never felt so alone in those last moments, in the midst of all those people.*' On the night the author's grandmother died, her two middle-aged daughters joined her in the bed, one on either side. One cannot know if this was a peaceful death or if even here there was no escaping that existential aloneness to which Keizer refers. But if grandmother *was* conscious of their presence she must have felt this warmth reaching out. And for these two sisters, there was a comforting meaning here: grandmother had, quite literally, died in her daughters' arms. The point here is that while on a *personal* and experiential level one dies alone, on an *interpersonal* or relational level we who are there must never withdraw our true presence.

---

**Reflective exercise 4.5: Confronting destiny**
**Time: 50 minutes**

Kubler-Ross[25] refers to a peaceful death. Keizer[26] speaks of the possibility of a less pleasant demise.

- Think for a moment about how you may eventually approach your own death.
- What feelings does an awareness that your time left is finite conjure up in you?

You cannot really know in advance *how* you will feel when the time comes. But are you aware of any beliefs or outlooks on life you hold that may influence how you will cope with this inevitable event?

- Reflect upon the extent to which you may have wanted to avoid this exercise or indeed found it unpleasant.
- Why is it that we avoid death as a topic in our culture? And why do we hide the dying from sight and sanitise the process of dying, death and bereavement?
- You may find it helpful to discuss these reflections with a colleague or friend, and ask them to share *their* views. But do remember to be sensitive – in our modern culture some people find it very distressing to even contemplate this topic.

## Conclusion

This chapter has no well-structured arguments, and no proposed formulae for the resolution of issues. Its sole purpose is to call the reader to reflect upon the experience of being seriously ill and perhaps even progressing to the terminal stages of illness and death. How we might respond to those living through such experience is an issue for other chapters in the book.

We have nevertheless attempted to consider the experience of illness in something of an orderly fashion. There are reflections on the nature of experience in illness, and there is an attempt to separate out the illness experience and the related disease process. We recognise also that each person's experience of illness and the journey through serious illness to recovery or death is unique. The journey metaphor allows us to recognise some of the aspects of this journey, from awareness and realisation, through the experience of suffering and the loneliness of this, to our seeking after meaning and – sometimes, though not always – coming to terms with how we might live through illness and eventually confront death.

But what do we now make of all this? Perhaps the most important point is this. The next time we walk the hospital ward or visit the sick room, and view the trappings of modern clinical technology and those appended to them, let us also remember that there are souls in the shadows. This heart is failing, and that cancer is growing, and we must of course respond to this knowledge. But it is the person (however we term this living presence – a soul, a being, a psyche) who feels the pain, experiences the misery and despair, and gazes out at us, perhaps imploringly. It is only if we gaze back as person to person that we can hope to achieve any understanding of what it is like to be where they are. We will never have a full understanding, not at least until our turn inevitably comes around. But we must believe that they see in *our* gaze that we care; that even as they eventually depart, in the words of songwriter Lucinda Williams,[27] we call after them this, as a hope rather than a question:

> *Did an angel whisper in your ear*
> *And hold you close and take away your fear*
> *In those long last moments.*

## References

1  Nouwen H. *In Memoriam*. Notre Dame, Indiana: Ave Maria Press; 1980, p. 26.
2  Fitzpatrick R. Lay concepts of illness. In: Fitzpatrick R, Hinton J, Newman S *et al.*, editors. *The Experience of Illness*. London: Tavistock Publications; 1984.
3  Sontag S. *Illness as Metaphor*. London: Penguin; 1983.
4  Sontag S. *AIDS and its Metaphors*. London: Penguin; 1990.
5  Cassell EJ. Treating patients for both is the healer's art: illness and disease. *Hastings Center Report*. 1976; **6**: 27–37.
6  Parsons T. *The Social System*. New York: Free Press; 1951.
7  Stockwell F. *The Unpopular Patient*. London: Royal College of Nursing; 1972.
8  Illich I. *Medical Nemesis: the expropriation of health*. New York: Pantheon; 1976.
9  Foucault M. *The Birth of the Clinic*. London: Tavistock; 1976.
10 Szasz T. *The Myth of Mental Illness*. London: Paladin; 1962.
11 Frank A. *The Wounded Storyteller: body, illness and ethics*. Chicago: University of Chicago Press; 1995.
12 Heidegger M. *Being and Time*. Oxford: Basil Blackwell Ltd; 1962.

13  Young J. Death and authenticity. In: Malpas J, Solomon RS, editors. *Death and Philosophy*. New York: Routledge; 1998, p. 112.

14  Elias N. *The Loneliness of the Dying*. New York: Continuum; 2001.

15  Morse JM. Towards a praxis theory of suffering. In: Cutcliffe J, McKenna H, editors. *The Essential Concepts of Nursing*. Edinburgh: Elsevier Churchill Livingstone; 2005.

16  O'Connor T. Agent causation. In: O'Connor T, editor. *Agents, Causes, and Events: essays on indeterminism and free will*. New York: Oxford University Press; 2003.

17  Gilbert P. What is shame? Some core issues and controversies. In: Gilbert P, Andrews B, editors. *Shame: interpersonal behaviour, psychopathology, and culture*. Oxford: Oxford University Press; 1998.

18  Groopman J. *The Anatomy of Hope: how people prevail in the face of illness*. New York: Random House; 2004.

19  Nouwen H. *The Wounded Healer*. London: Darton, Longman and Todd; 1994.

20  Kearney M. *Mortally Wounded: stories of soul pain, death and healing*. Dublin: Marino Books; 1996.

21  Slevin O. Spirituality and nursing. In: Basford L, Slevin O, editors. *Theory and Practice of Nursing: an integrated approach to caring practice*, 2nd edition. Cheltenham: Nelson Thornes; 2003.

22  Hillman J. *A Blue Fire*. New York: Harper Perennial; 1991.

23  Cheng C. Onto-epistemology of sudden enlightenment in Chan Buddhism. *Chung-Hua Buddhist Journal*. 2000; **13**(2): 585–611.

24  Frankl V. *Man's Search for Meaning*. New York: Washington Square Press; 1985.

25  Kubler-Ross E. *On Death and Dying*. London: Tavistock; 1969.

26  Keizer B. *Dancing with Mister D: notes on life and death*. London: Doubleday; 1996.

27  Williams L. Lake Charles. On: Williams L. *Car Wheels on a Gravel Road* [CD]. New York: Mercury Records/Warner-Tamerlane Pub. Corp; 1998.

# Complementary chapters

*See also Stepping into Palliative Care 1: relationships and responses*

- Chapter 3: The cancer journey
- Chapter 5: The psychological impact of serious illness
- Chapter 6: Hope and coping strategies
- Chapter 7: The therapeutic relationship
- Chapter 15: Transcultural and ethnic issues at the end of life
- Chapter 16: Sexuality and palliative care

*See also Stepping into Palliative Care 2: care and practice*

- Chapter 9: The last few days of life
- Chapter 11: Breaking bad news
- Chapter 12: Hearing the pain of the carer
- Chapter 13: Spirituality and palliative care
- Chapter 14: Bereavement

# Chapter 5

# The psychological impact of serious illness

*Phil Barker and Poppy Buchanan-Barker*

---

**Pre-reading exercise 5.1**
**Time: 20 minutes**

You are sitting on the edge of your bed awaiting the results of your scan. The nurse is fumbling with your notes. The doctor kneels beside you and smiles, touching you gently on the arm. He says that he will speak to a colleague in the morning but 'It's not looking too good. Maybe we should be prepared for the worst'.

- You wonder – 'What does he mean *we*?'
- Use your imagination. How do you *feel*?

---

## Introduction

Palliative care – as the name implies – aims to ameliorate the symptoms or effects of almost any illness, but typically is focused on the more serious end of the illness spectrum.

### Serious illness

Serious illnesses come in all disguises. By *serious* we mean 'life-threatening' or at least 'life-disrupting'. Most illnesses have the potential to threaten or disrupt our lives if left untreated or when someone is already weakened constitutionally.

However, some illnesses are more threatening than others. Some arrive suddenly, swiftly and dramatically, changing our whole sense of ourselves and our mortality. Others steal slowly into our lives, subtly changing one thing after another, almost unnoticed, under our very noses. We awaken, one morning, to the realisation that we are not the person we once were. Others set alarm bells ringing when they first appear, then recede, but continue to gnaw away, quietly but relentlessly; eroding our abilities, draining our confidence, sapping our *joie de vivre*. However intermittent, or in the background, these too are serious in their effects on our lives.

We shall focus here on the psychological impact of serious illness: what it means in the context of the person's life. Illness is a human construct and its experience is a human problem. However, the 'psychological distress' associated with illness is often not clearly articulated.[1]

The *experiences* associated with, for example, progressive difficulty in swallowing, undergoing tests and examinations, and ultimately receiving a diagnosis of oeso-phageal cancer, are psychological. By this we mean such experiences are expressed through the person's *thoughts*, *feelings* and associated *beliefs*. Such experiences are deeply personal. How could they be otherwise?

Often it is very difficult to find out what, exactly, is happening for the person – at least through direct questioning. This reminds us that, rather than seeking precise answers to our questions about care and treatment, palliative care focuses on 'personal responses': what needs to be done! Considering the palliative care of people who are dying, Roy[2] recognised that the communication of needs can be very subtle:

> *Often the questions themselves cannot really be spoken about. If we are listening only for words, we may well miss questions and quests that dying people are trying to show us, and we will miss showing them the response, the absence of which is the cause of their suffering.*[2]

## Being people-friendly

We shall discuss the psychological impact of serious illness in plain language. Much psychology might be described as 'everything we ever knew, in language we do not understand!' Given its inherent human nature we shall try to respect the ways by which people, in our experience, typically think and feel about their experience of illness, pain or suffering. Respecting their way of *talking* about thoughts and feelings is the first step in respecting the person. It is also the first step towards understanding how we might help them address their suffering.

## Bothered by illness and bewildered by medicine

The expropriation of the *experience* of illness – and its associated *suffering* – was one of the first motives of medicine. *Suffering* refers to the experience of 'being required to undergo' some form of pain or difficulty, whether physical, emotional or spiritual. It may be no accident that medicine, and to some extent psychology, distanced itself from 'suffering' by focusing on the putative 'causes' or 'processes' of illness, in an attempt to develop an 'objective science'.

Medicine developed its own special language to describe both the body and the various disorders that might afflict it. Psychology followed suit, developing its own private language of 'mind' and 'person'. In so doing, it dispossessed people of their direct *experience*, rendering their natural descriptions inferior, if not redundant.

## The value of humility

Illness is a naturally disempowering force. People know what it is like to 'struggle for breath' and most find their own metaphors to describe the experience. Renaming this – *dyspnoea* or *apnoea* – does not advance the person's understanding of what is happening. Often, such language merely disempowers them further, as they are blinded by the language of medicine.

One of our first responsibilities in palliative care is to return the 'power of story' to the person. To do so, we need to acquire a degree of humility, so that we might learn from the person who is suffering.

## The person's experience

### What is happening to me?

All people are psychologically complex – some more than others. Some smile and nod agreeably as we inform them about a forthcoming examination or operation. Others fight back tears, stare blankly, become angry, or even appear indifferent. *Why* people react in one way or another is worthy of a chapter itself. For now we would suggest there is a value in *not knowing* why.

Because we are all human, we assume that we can understand what is happening, emotionally, for another person. We might call it sympathy, empathy or fellow feeling. All suggest a deeply felt recognition *and* understanding of someone else's experience. We risk saying 'Yes, I *know* how you feel' when clearly we can never know another person's experience.

Indeed, there is a danger that such fellow feeling will be counterproductive. By feeling too much for the person we may prevent them from connecting, more deeply, with their own thoughts and feelings; making more sense of their suffering. Striking the right balance between not feeling enough for people and feeling too much is no easy matter. Like all human qualities necessary to care for *people* this can only be acquired through experience.

Often it is better to accept that we have no idea about what is happening for the person. Then we might ask, simply and with genuine curiosity:

- 'How do you feel about that?' or
- 'What do you think of that?'

The person is trying to 'make sense' of all that is happening to them – *privately*, as they examine their own thoughts and feelings, and *publicly*, as they talk with and listen to members of the care team. 'Making sense' lies at the heart of the psychology of the experience of illness. Any help the professional team might offer involves no more than elaborations on this natural 'sense making'. All we can do is help the person clarify the meaning of their experience, personally. There are no psychological 'techniques' or 'tricks' to help people 'feel better'. All we can hope for is that we might help the person grow to some new understanding of themselves and their illness.

### Vulnerability

Arguably, the commonest experience among people who are seriously ill is vulnerability. This term has various definitions in the professional literature or the dictionary. All suggest the potential to suffer harm or hurt, whether physical or psychological. However, what does vulnerability mean in lay terms – for the person?

- What do they *experience* when vulnerable?
- What happens, *as a result* – whether directly or indirectly – of those experiences?

Such meanings are like stones, cast into a pool. Their ripples touch others far removed from the action: family or friends and especially those intimately involved in caring for the person – the professional team members. Vulnerability talks to and touches everyone.

A host of situations can herald vulnerability. When people are ill, especially but not exclusively in hospital, they are dressed in nightwear and dressing gowns, traditionally as a medical convenience, to allow ease of examination. Stripped of our day clothes, wearing attire that may be as revealing as it is unfashionable, we feel vulnerable. We are embarrassed and self-conscious. This feeling may pass, as we habituate to the situation, but our status as a person has been diminished and will need some rehabilitation.

*'Becoming a patient'* can be an emotional watershed. The institutional structure of healthcare – whether in hospital wards, community clinics or the patient's own home – often places people at a disadvantage. Professionals often exercise this advantage over patients as an unconscious way of dealing with their own anxieties.[3] This might involve anxiety over their limited skill or knowledge, or anxiety concerning their feelings about the patient's plight. Regrettably, practitioners are often unaware of the extent to which they 'defend' themselves against these anxieties: by being bossy, aloof, inappropriately humorous, stern or 'professionally distant'. Any of these strategies may heighten the patient's sense of vulnerability and hinder the development of the close, confiding relationship that is so obviously desired – and necessary.

The person's vulnerability triggers other feelings. Among these are fears that they will:

- appear *foolish*, by asking questions about their illness or treatment – thereby displaying their ignorance
- be *judged*, especially if they believe (rightly or wrongly) that their illness is a result of their lifestyle, or genetic make-up
- be *'kept in the dark'* over their condition, its seriousness, treatment or likely development
- be *exploited*, physically, emotionally or even financially, because they are, temporarily, weakened by illness
- become *'public knowledge'*, now that their story is known and discussed by so many different people
- be *neglected* by staff, whom they believe are minimising their concerns or appear to be complacent over their plight.

## Meaning and metaphor

The greatest vulnerability is *not having needs met*. All too often care and treatment focuses on the illness, in its various physical manifestations, as if unrelated to the person who is ill. It is not necessary to involve complex, abstract theories or models of 'holistic care'. We need only accept that every ache or pain, every procedure administered, every kilogram lost or scar gained, is experienced by the person. The person is the captain of the ship of life and is logging every detail of the voyage through illness. There is much to learn from this intrepid sailor.

We introduce this sea-faring metaphor to remind the reader that much of what people experience, when in pain or otherwise ill, is beyond words. Or at least, often no words can be readily found that seem fitting or appropriate. This is why we all have recourse to metaphor: the pain is *stabbing* or *burning* – or the person feels as if they are being stabbed, or burnt. These metaphors have found their way into pain questionnaires, for example. However, although we might have helpful metaphors of our own, we should be curious to discover how the person would describe their own experience: what metaphors do they choose?

Even where the team members are highly sophisticated, they should not assume that they *know* what the person's needs are. Although there are many occasions where it is necessary, indeed vital, that the professional 'take charge', we risk sidelining the person if we do not try to 'care with', as well as caring *for* and caring *about* them. We 'care with' by trying to clarify, through open conversation, *what* needs to be done and *why*. Sometimes, people will ask for things that are beyond our capabilities or immediate resources or even are unethical. We gain the person's confidence if, at least, we allow them to make their needs or wishes known to us. And so, their vulnerability begins to diminish.

## Growing from anguish to meaning

In palliative care meaning is, quite literally, *vital*. People are meaning-makers. We dedicate much of our lives to making sense of *who* we are: as individuals and family members, friends or lovers. At the same time we try to make sense of *what* we do in our lives that is meaning*ful*, and we bemoan the presence of the meaning*less*. Professionals with a highly developed knowledge of the body, its workings and associated afflictions risk forgetting that suffering is about meaning, not physiology. People can endure great pain and torment if it has 'a point' or personal meaning. Viktor Frankl, the psychiatrist who survived the experience of four Nazi concentration camps, reminded us that: 'Man [*sic*] is not destroyed by suffering, he is destroyed by suffering without meaning.'[4]

## Classic stages

Where illness is life-threatening, people appear to move through discrete stages or phases, displaying changing responses to their plight and often those around them. Table 5.1 illustrates some classic understandings of the stages of what might be called 'psychic pain'. Often described as 'mourning' or 'grief' reactions, these refer to what is being lost through the process of serious, life-threatening illness.

Table 5.1 Psychological dimensions of life-threatening illness

| Stages[5] | Phases[6] | Reactions[7] |
|---|---|---|
| Denial | Shock, numbness, disbelief | 'No, this can't be happening to me' |
| Emergence of emotions, especially anger | Feelings of guilt, anger, sadness, resentment | 'Why me, why now?' |
| Bargaining | Yearning, searching, pining | 'Yes, this is happening to me but ...' |
| Depression | Grieving | 'Yes, this is happening' |
| Acceptance | Resolution | 'Yes' |

Although useful in a general sense, these 'models' can be ill-fitting where the story of one individual is concerned, who may take a different course through their suffering. This should be interesting rather than problematic. We can learn so much about 'what is happening' for this *particular person*, by listening carefully to their 'expert' story.

Whenever we become ill we begin a private dialogue, which focuses on exploring and hopefully understanding what is 'happening' within our being. In the early stages of serious illness, the person might ask:

- *Concern* – Why can't I swallow properly?
- *Worry* – Is there something wrong with me?
- *Indecision* – Should I have this checked or wait and see what happens?

Later, the person might wrestle with a very different set of questions:

- *Anger* – Why did this happen to me?
- *Regret* – Why didn't I get this checked earlier?
- *Hopelessness* – Why is nothing working?

All such questions focus on a search for meaning. Even when no solution can be found – for the pain, discomfort or fear – glimmers of meaning can act as a psychic balm, easing the person's suffering.

## Scary reflections

The person who is grieving or mourning the effects of their illness is likely to reflect on the life they have lived and the life ahead, which may well be denied them. They may be asking:

- What have I done with my life?
- What kind of a person have I been?
- What has my life meant for my family and friends?
- What do my family and friends think of me, now?
- What is important for me now?

How the person addresses these various questions – or their assorted emotional consequences – depends very much on the kind of person they have become, through their life experience. We often talk about people's ability to *cope* with illness, suffering, or impending death. 'Coping' is a catch-all expression, referring to all sorts of private, invisible actions the person might take in responding to their situation.

How people respond to difficult circumstances depends on a wide range of factors. These include the extent to which they:

- feel supported, by family or friends
- are able to communicate, openly and constructively, with others
- are able, and willing, to access and talk about their feelings, especially their fears and anxieties
- have spiritual beliefs and have reflected on their own mortality
- are concerned for the welfare of others, and how *they* will cope with their death and its various consequences.

Serious illness brings all manner of losses in its wake. At some point the person will look in the mirror of their everyday experience and realise what, exactly, has been lost – never to be returned. Common losses are:

- *Health* – I am losing my strength, vigour and physical dynamism.
- *Capability* – I am no longer able to do all the things I used to be able to do.
- *Self-concept* – I am beginning to feel differently about myself. Who am I becoming?
- *Aesthetics* – I am old, ugly, damaged or repulsive.
- *Functionality* – My leg, arm, mind (etc.) just won't work the way it once did.
- *Independence* – I am becoming reliant on others. This is a new experience.
- *Social* – Who will come and see me *now*?
- *Occupation* – Will I ever work again? What have I to offer the world?

In addition, the person may also begin to appreciate the importance of everyday activities, which they have largely taken for granted:

- reading
- gardening
- walking the dog
- taking breakfast in a favourite café
- having a drink with a friend after work
- shopping, anonymously, in a large supermarket
- buying a book from a bookstore.

The list of such 'activity losses' is endless. As the staff efficiently glide through their hospice routines, or drive to a home visit, the person is likely to be scanning through their growing catalogue of loss.

Forming a backdrop to this 'activity loss list' stand other, more general, but no less disabling, losses:

- concentration
- sleep
- social status
- family role
- financial security
- personal identity
- satisfaction
- sense of achievement.

Serious illness provides a mirror of the soul, sharper and more penetrating than any other reflection we have encountered. Where the person believes that this is the final chapter of their life story, the reflection may be humbling, humiliating or disarming. The person amounts to nothing more than a collection of memories, some good, some full of regret. They may feel angry at a life about to be cut short, or sorrowful at their many missed opportunities, of a life not 'fully lived'. They may feel ashamed at their inability to show or accept love and friendship. They may feel guilt over wrongdoings – whether real or imagined.

# Professional responses

This complex scenario suggests that professional care must be equally complex and unfathomable. Paradoxically, this is not the case. All that the professional need do is:

- provide some *encouragement* – helping the person express their feelings, openly, without fear of rejection. We cannot value enough the importance of '*feeling in control, being able to say things to loved ones, feeling at peace with world, being able to express openly emotions without being judged, whether displaying anger, joy, love or fear*'[8]
- *normalise* the experience – pain and suffering are the commonest of human experiences. What they signify – defect, decay and eventually death – will be common to everyone, eventually. Pregnancy and birth are not 'diseases' or 'pathology' but a part of healthy living. Mortality is also a part of life. Why should we pathologise it? Why should people not experience a 'healthy' death?

## Facing loss

Confronting loss is rarely easy. Where the person has valued highly certain qualities in their lifetime – for example, looks, intelligence or fitness – losing them will be doubly difficult. Such losses may also resonate strongly with members of the care team who begin to wonder how they will feel when they (inevitably) begin to decline – aesthetically, intellectually or dynamically.

The mutuality of such experiences – something that will be shared, ultimately, by everyone – should make talk about deterioration and the likelihood of death easier. Paradoxically, the knowledge that we all will wither and die seems to deter discussion, prompting denial of our own mortality. Such denial prevents us from connecting with the person. It also reminds us of the need for all healthcare professionals to be helped to talk, openly, about *their* feelings about illness and death.

## Facing death

We can never experience our death, but can only experience life. People may imagine their death, but such imaginings remain part of their 'lived experience'. Is it too optimistic to suggest that dying can be an opportunity for human development? We think not, and know several people, personally, who grew remarkably, as persons, into the very jaws of death. Dying can be an undignified affair, with all manner of clamour and caterwauling – whether from family or overstretched professional teams. However, if people can be afforded a dignified exit from this life, the final stages of their voyage might bring new insights, or allow the healing of old wounds. It might even be a cause for celebration rather than just a 'blessed release'.

People might grow into the final stages of life if they can:

- complete their necessary 'worldly affairs'
- conclude their personal and professional relationships
- learn something of the 'meaning of life'
- come to love themselves and those who are important to them
- accept the finality of life and the inevitability of death
- sense a new 'self' beyond the self that is, slowly, being lost

- recognise a transcendent realm
- give themselves up to the unknown.[9]

For us, these various 'actions' – many of them vague and mysterious if not mystical – can contribute to a physical sense of peace. Are these the ultimate tasks of life? Has our life been no more than a rehearsal for these steps into the emptiness of the great beyond, or the Path to Enlightenment or Heaven, whichever is our favoured belief? Who knows?

What is important is that people are helped to complete these tasks. These are not about dying – but are about completing the complex business of living.

## Meaningful care

Although everyone is unique, as human beings we are all more alike than different. In that human sense, some common principles can be established, concerning human problems and how we might respond to them.

Specific fears commonly heighten our sense of suffering. As Copp's classic study showed,[10] most patients experience:

- fear of *anticipated* pain
- fear of being *alone*
- fear of the *unknown*
- fear of *procedures* and *equipment*.

The resourceful professional can, with a little ingenuity and creativity, develop ways of addressing each of these fears – ideally through discussion and negotiation with the person.

## Conclusion

People may begin their voyage into the stormy and dangerous waters of serious illness with the assumption that we – the professional caregivers – will rescue them. Soon they will learn what, exactly, professional care can offer. Often they will realise that what is on offer is sorely limited. However, this does not mean that it is not of great human value.

Hopefully, people also come to appreciate the lessons in living that illness has to offer. They may also discover what they, personally, can bring to the encounter, or their battle with Fate.

## Need for supervision

Similar lessons exist for all members of the care team, but especially those required to spend long periods in intimate contact with patients and their families, hearing their stories about the meaning of illness. Working with seriously ill people, especially those confronting death, can be a heart-rending occupation.

Some staff choose this area of work in the expectation that it will, in time, become meaningful for them. For them the occupation is more of a vocation or perhaps personal voyage. All staff, however, need to be carefully supported to allow the development of the 'moral imagination' so necessary to palliative care.[11] Life-threatening illness is a profound human experience, not just for patients but for all in any way concerned. Sensitive, skilled supervision is needed to allow practitioners to express some of their own psychic struggles with the experience of caring,[12] so that they can continue to face their own mortality, reflected in the eyes of the patient.

---

**Reflective exercise 5.1**
**Time: 20 minutes**

*Recall* a time when you were 'suffering' – experiencing physical or emotional pain. Or recall a time when your life was disrupted through a temporary loss of everyday function – broken limb, loss of energy, or lengthy confinement in bed.

- List the feelings you had *then*.

*Imagine* that your 'suffering' was to last 'indefinitely', or was a sign of something worse to come.

- List the feelings you are having *now*.

---

# References

1   Rider SH. Psychological distress: concept analysis. *Journal of Advanced Nursing*. 2004; **45**(5): 785–793.
2   Roy DJ. Palliative care: a fragment towards a philosophy of palliative care. *Journal of Palliative Care*. 1997; **13**(1): 3–4.
3   Menzies-Lyth I. The functions of social systems as a defence against anxiety: a report on a study of the nursing service of a general hospital. *Human Relations*. 1959; **13**: 95–121.
4   Frankl VE. *Man's Search for Meaning*. New York: Simon and Schuster; 1984.
5   Kubler-Ross E. *On Death and Dying*. London: Tavistock Publications; 1969.
6   Parkes CM. *Studies of Grief in Adult Life*. Harmondsworth: Pelican; 1972.
7   Bowlby J. Loss: sadness and depression. In: Bowlby, J. *Attachment and Loss*, 3rd edition. Harmondsworth: Penguin; 1981.
8   Russell P, Sander R. Palliative care: promoting the concept of a healthy death. *British Journal of Nursing*. 1998; **7**(5): 256–261.
9   Byock IR. *Dying Well: the prospect of growth at the end of life*. New York: Riverhead/Putnam Books; 1997.
10  Copp LA. The spectrum of suffering. *American Journal of Nursing*. 1990; **8**: 35–39.
11  Georges JJ, Grypdonck M, De Casterle BD. Being a palliative care nurse in an academic hospital: a qualitative study about nurses' perception of palliative care nursing. *Journal of Clinical Nursing*. 2002; **11**(6): 785–793.
12  Jones A. Out of sight – an existential-phenomenology method of clinical supervision: the contribution to palliative care. *Journal of Advanced Nursing*. 1998; **27**(5): 905–913.

# To learn more

- Langer TS. *Choices for Living: coping with fear of dying*. New York: Springer; 2002.
- Snyder CR, Lopez SJ. *Handbook of Positive Psychology*. New York: Oxford University Press; 2001.
- Turner J, Kelly B. The concept of debriefing and its application to staff dealing with life-threatening illnesses such as cancer, AIDS and other conditions. In: Raphael B, Wilson JP. *Psychological Debriefing: theory, practice and evidence*. Cambridge: Cambridge University Press; 2000, Chapter 18.

# Complementary chapters

*See also Stepping into Palliative Care 1: relationships and responses*

- Chapter 2: What is palliative care?
- Chapter 3: The cancer journey
- Chapter 4: The experience of illness
- Chapter 6: Hope and coping strategies
- Chapter 7: The therapeutic relationship
- Chapter 12: Stress issues in palliative care

*See also Stepping into Palliative Care 2: care and practice*

- Chapter 11: Breaking bad news
- Chapter 12: Hearing the pain of the carer
- Chapter 13: Spirituality and palliative care

# Hope and coping strategies

*Jo Cooper and David B Cooper*

## Coping strategies

*Coping: A process by which a person deals with stress, solves problems and makes decisions ...*[1]

---

**Reflective exercise 6.1**
**Time: 20 minutes**

Consider and reflect on:

- What do you think the person with a diagnosis of cancer has to cope with? *Include physical, psychological, emotional and spiritual elements.*
- What do you think their fears might include?
- How do you cope in times of difficulty?

Compare your feelings with your answers.

- Do they differ?
- If so, how?

---

Following a diagnosis of cancer, people face the enormous challenge of a threat to their existence and may use many different and varied approaches to reduce emotional distress. Each individual travels a unique life journey. The way in which we cope with illness depends on past experiences, characteristics and personality. Each person responds differently to difficulties and copes in his or her individual way.

Although there are different strategies to aid coping, four primary psychological responses have been identified[2] that can be grouped into four themes (*see* Figure 6.1):

1 denial
2 fighting spirit
3 acceptance
4 hopelessness.

When dealing with coping strategies, it is essential to remember that the concept of coping is a dynamic and fluctuating process[3] and people use a range of coping strategies, dependent on the situation. It is important not to permanently place the person into any one coping strategy, as each individual is unique in their response and attitudes may change over time.

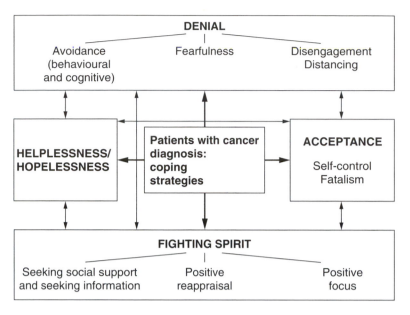

**Figure 6.1**   Patients with cancer diagnosis – coping strategies.

## Denial and acceptance as coping strategies

Case scenario 6.1

Jen (51) was in the late stages of metastatic breast cancer. It had spread to her bones and liver, despite aggressive chemotherapy. She was married to Jim, and had two teenage sons. Her mother had died 2 years previously with lung cancer, and had experienced a painful death from bone metastases. Jen began having vivid, powerful and unpleasant dreams. These centred on the destructive elements of her illness, her loss of control and her fear of becoming a burden to her family, particularly her husband. Jen was distressed by her dreams and felt confused and muddled by their content. There was no order to them and she was unable to verbalise any of her fears and feelings to her family. She was trying to protect them from her own fears. Jen was trying to cope with the inevitable losses that she was facing.

Reflective exercise 6.2
Time: 15 minutes

Consider and reflect on:

• How would you help Jen cope with her intense feelings and muddled thoughts?

## Helping Jen explore her story

The key skill required when helping Jen is *listening* to her story.

- Listen to her fears.
- Observe her body expression.
- Ask simple, explorative, questions:
    - How do you feel about ...?
    - How are you coping with ...?
    - What happens to you when you feel that you can't cope?

This will encourage Jen to think and reflect on her difficulties and explore how she is feeling and coping. By *attentive listening* you will understand:

- how Jen is coping
- what she is struggling to cope with.

It is important to acknowledge Jen's distress, grief and difficulties, so that Jen knows she has been *heard*. Feeling listened to and being supported is a powerful vehicle in the maintenance of coping.

---

**Key tip 6.1**

- Practical problems do not always have practical solutions.
- It does not matter if we do not have the answers.
- The answer is in the help and support that we can give.

---

## Helping Jen

Because Jen found it hard initially to say how she was feeling, she was encouraged to paint what she saw in her dreams. She did this at home, using simple watercolours. This helped to give some order and structure to her thoughts, making it easier to explore and verbalise them. She was able to talk through her pictures, deciphering for herself each theme and the meaning it had for her. Over several weeks, Jen made some sense of her feelings and felt able speak freely about her fears. Through gradual progression Jen discovered:

- she was fearful of losing her family by being a burden to them
- loss of body integrity – she felt overweight and ugly
- loss of her mother and her own fear of a painful death
- loss of independence – her job as a director and her loss of status
- loss of her role as a mother and being denied the joys and sorrows of watching her children mature into adulthood
- loss of sexual intimacy with her husband
- realisation that she was coping by denying her death and the effect this had on her and the family.

## What about Jen's family?

Including Jen's family in discussions around their own fears, and how they were coping, was important. This not only helped and nurtured them, but supported Jen in knowing that her family felt supported.

## Acceptance and action

Jen slowly began to accept the inevitability of her death but occasionally used denial to create some normality in her life. She planned a family holiday for the summer (*hope*), but was also able to talk with Jim about the realities of their situation, and plan her funeral, choosing the hymns and the music. However, Jen remained unable to talk to her sons, other than superficially.

There could be an assumption here that once acceptance has been achieved, this is permanent and stable.[4] However, generally this is not the case.[5,6] People who are dying may use denial as a sole defence or they may exhibit elements of partial denial at different times during the dying process. Often partial denial is used, fluctuating with acceptance, as in Jen's situation.

## So is denial good or bad?

Denial, avoidance and distancing are ways of providing self-deception, protecting the person from stress.[7] This buys time and allows the individual to have periods of normality. It is important to explore denial, in case it is concealing psychological distress, as it was for Jen. An *area of uncertain certainty* exists between open acknowledgement of death and the desire to deny it.[8] This has been termed *middle knowledge*, and can occur at critical transition stages – for example, when a person experiences setbacks or descends towards death.[4] Therefore, the person:

- has accepted the facts of their illness
- is facing imminent death
- but has the need to occasionally resist the finite nature of their situation.[4]

---

**Reflective exercise 6.3**
**Time: 20 minutes**

Consider and reflect on the following:

- Have you witnessed people using denial?
- How did you view denial then?
- Have you felt, or been told by another professional, that denial is a negative coping strategy?
- What are your thoughts on denial now?

---

## What can I do?

Denial, as a coping strategy, can be a source of concern to the professional. Historically, denial has been viewed as a negative method of coping. It has been felt that people, in order to accept their situation realistically, should be prepared to discuss sensitive issues around their death. However, not everyone wants to openly acknowledge their illness, its implications and their death, and they should be given the right to choose whether or not to disclose.

Talking about dying is not communicated as a single encounter, more as a series of interactions with patients and families which nurture understanding, acceptance and coping over time.[9] Open communication takes time and skill. The professional is led by the patient as to what s/he wishes to disclose. Helping the individual to uncover his or her feelings and fears is important in maintaining mental wellbeing. Negative feelings, such as anger and fear, *can be helped*.

# Fighting spirit as a coping strategy

> **Case scenario 6.2**
>
> John (66) was diagnosed with advanced lung cancer. Supportive treatment in terms of symptomatic relief was offered. John had no family and lived in a hostel for people with drug and alcohol problems. He had little in life, no family or material assets, but he felt he had *everything* to live for, and wanted to survive.

## *Exploring John's story*

John accepted the full implications of his illness and accepted the fact that he would die (acceptance). However, at the same time John was determined to *fight*.

He would say, '*I won't let the cancer beat me, I'll try everything to get better ... I want to make it to my 70th birthday ...*' – and on another day, '*I've had a good life ... what is left is a bonus*'.

## *Maintaining hope*

John was able to maintain a positive outlook and viewed his cancer as a challenge. His attitude was optimistic and he generally had very little distress. Initially, his hope was that the future would bring a *miracle cure*, or that the doctors had *got it wrong* (*false hope*). However, over time, as John deteriorated, his hope (*realistic hope*) was for a death without pain. John began to accept the inevitability of his death. He confided that he hoped that he would not be judged for what he described as *leading an amoral life*.

John's coping strategy of fighting spirit enabled him to cope with life stresses, protecting against fears and anxieties. He was not overwhelmed by distress, even though this was not entirely absent. He wanted information and support and engaged in open communication about his situation.

# Hopelessness as a coping strategy

---

**Case scenario 6.3**

Sarah (58) was diagnosed with oesophageal cancer. Despite chemotherapy and the offer of substantial professional and family support, she felt over-whelmed by her situation. She was immobilised by her circumstances and unable to make any effort to cope or adjust and abandoned hope from the outset. Her family felt that she had everything to live for. She had a devoted husband, Peter, two adult daughters, a large house, and was financially secure. She and Peter holidayed abroad twice a year; they kept horses and she taught disabled children to ride. Although Sarah accepted chemotherapy, she felt that it was futile. She was unable to talk about her fears or concerns and was anxious and depressed, a sense of hopelessness contributing to the development of depression. Sarah became dependent on her family and did not actively seek knowledge or information about her condition.

---

## Helping Sarah

To the professional and others caring for Sarah it felt as though she was unhelpable, leaving them with a sense of helplessness; mirroring some of Sarah's own feelings.

---

**Reflective exercise 6.4**
**Time: 15 minutes**

Consider and reflect on:

- Why do you think Sarah felt hopeless?
- What would you do to enable a less traumatic situation for Sarah?

---

It is not unusual for individuals using this coping strategy to *give up*.[10] Sarah chose never to disclose her fears: only to say that she perceived her cancer as a punishment and expressed a loss of hope in her future. She blamed herself for her illness and felt guilty when her treatment failed. However, the role of the professional is one of enabling – looking towards how blame is attributed, and directing interventions towards correcting misconceptions. There may have been instances whereby lifestyle had contributed to the cause of cancer. It is only by listening that we can begin to help, smoothing the way forward. The role is one of facilitation and exploration and the art and skill of professional practice is about supporting as things become difficult.[11,12]

We cannot change events for Sarah. It is difficult to know how to promote hope in a person close to death. However, respecting individuality can help to facilitate hope.[12] This may activate positive coping, leading to a stable sense of wellbeing.

# Assessing, approaching and caring

Ongoing assessment and review of coping behaviours and their impact on the individual and family is cardinal in enabling compassionate and understanding care and attention. If provision of care and attention is to be humane, compassionate and perceptive, then listening and responding are pivotal skills. However, ongoing assessment and review must go hand in hand as essential components to approaching and caring.

It is uncertain whether maintaining hope in the face of advanced disease is a form of denial or a distinct coping strategy in itself.[9] Hopes for the future are an integral part of our emotional wellbeing, whether or not we are experiencing illness. However, the need to maintain hope influences the amount of information sought and is an important strategy in helping people to cope with the knowledge of their disease.[9]

# Hope

Above we have looked at the various coping strategies we use; here we turn to how the professional can enable *hope*.

## What is hope?

Hope is at the centre of our being and spirit. It can be our:

- religion
- story or journey
- love of nature
- trust of a friend
- precious moment in time.

Hope is whatever is meaningful to us – whatever helps us cope with our illness and dis-ease. Hope is intertwined with goal achieving, which gives us some kind of reward and pleasure. Therefore, the professionals' role is pivotal to enable the individual to identify hope, and think about the possibilities.

## How do we enable hope?

Enabling (*facilitating*) hope is about identifying things in the present, goals to aim for that are achievable. To give false hope by identifying hope that is not practical or achievable is destructive. The professional, patient and family relationship must be open and honest, sharing what can be done, and what cannot be done. Hope is about considering possibilities.

Quintessentially, it is a waste of all we know to work in the insular belief that all individuals are the same. Therefore, it is pivotal to:

- *meet* the patient, family and your minds at the same point
- work *with* them to identify hope
- work *with* them to achieve their chosen goal(s) – hope.

Hope is at the heart of coping[13] and one can only hope if the goal is realistic. The key points of hope have been identified as follows:[13]

- Hope is a realistic desire for something good in the face of uncertainty.
- Hope is not about denial or optimism.

- Hope changes as the illness progresses.
- A trusted, listening ear is the most helpful support, not someone who offers false reassurance.

## So why is hope so important?

Hope has been described as:

> ... an inner power or strength that can enrich lives and enable individuals to look beyond their pain, suffering and turmoil ...[14]

Categories and sub-categories to hope-fostering and hope-hindering include the following.[11,12]

*Hope-fostering:*

- love of family and friends[14]
- spirituality/having faith[14]
- setting goals and maintaining independence[14]
- positive relationships with professionals[14]
- humour[14]/lightheartedness[12]
- personal characteristics[14]
- uplifting memories.[14]

*Hope-hindering:*

- abandonment and isolation[12,14]
- uncontrolled pain and discomfort[12,14]
- devaluation of personhood[12,14]
- inability to visualise any meaningful future.

## Bringing about exploration

Assessment is where the exploration of hope, and how it can be enabled, commences. It is a process of continual appraisal that is open to change and or abandonment as the identified needs dictate.

Hope is integral to the psychological needs and wellbeing of the patient and family. Understanding and enabling hope improves the quality of patient care, and life. Respect and courtesy[14] are important; conversely, poor communication and failure to acknowledge the needs of the individual are destructive and detrimental.

Therefore, *how* do we identify and explore hope? The following checklist might be useful:

- Identify events that might bring hope.
- Recognise problems in achieving hope that are likely to be experienced.
- Assist the individual(s) in the process of acknowledging, exploring and understanding barriers to hope.
- Appreciate the individual's perception of hope and its barriers.
- Consider together the options available.
- Facilitate the individual's achievement of the chosen goal (hope).
- Acquaint the individual(s) with services and facilities available to attain the goal (hope).

- Be non-judgmental.
- Provide maximum professional intervention.
- Provide maximum understanding and support.
- Keep to your word.
- Keep goals (hope) realistic and achievable.
- Explore what is and what is not achievable to avoid building false hope.
- Speak truthfully.
- Be open to possibilities.

Ask exploratory questions, e.g.:

- What does hope mean to you?
- Tell me about your hope. What sort of thing do you hope for?
- If you could identify a source of hope for yourself, what would it be?
- What things cause you to lose hope?
- What helps you to maintain hope or maybe makes you feel hopeful?[14]

## Where do we go from here?

Once the individual comes to a place in his or her mind where s/he can take charge of life, then the professional can encourage the move to action. The acceptance that hope does not mean a cure, or that all will be well, but that life is good regardless of the conclusion is a step forward. To achieve this, the professional needs to support the individual to a point where s/he can:

- identify where s/he is now and what expectation s/he has for the future
- acknowledge what the illness will bring
- take time to reflect on what s/he knows and does not know
- identify where support and care will come from and how to access this.

## Where do I come in?

A good starting point is to look at each day and explore what is necessary and what is achievable – this could be a simple task like shopping. It is helpful to assist the individual to concentrate on life as if it were *normal*: what would s/he usually do in terms of daily tasks or recreational activities. The emphasis is on what can still be done and not on what cannot be done. If the individual enjoys dancing or golf, while it may not be possible to fully participate as the illness progresses, it may be possible to slowly reduce the activity or participate from another perspective rather than stop altogether. It is not about giving up in anticipation of death but looking at maintaining the normality of life as long as possible and making gradual reductions to accommodate the illness.

## The family

People are able to deal with pain, loss of independence and relationships by maintaining hope. Having hope extends to the family as much as to the patient. For them, maintaining hope is important in terms of helping the patient to achieve each daily goal (hope) and for themselves to achieve their hope(s). To do that each family member needs to identify where s/he is in relation to self and the patient, working together in an environment where they can share worries, hopes, questions and answers. It is important for the family to understand and appreciate that they can offer something to their loved one, be that shopping with the individual, washing hair or, in the later stages of the illness, bathing or massaging.[11]

### Recognising that hope is there

Hope is difficult to describe. It means many things to many people, each having their own interpretation. However, it can be said that without hope there is no life. Life does not stop because one becomes ill; it merely changes the perspective on life and, with that, the individual needs to find a way to keep life rewarding until there is no life. Therefore by:

- being supportive and caring
- being *with* and meeting the patient and family at the point where they are
- keeping pain effectively managed
- openness
- developing trust
- exploring and developing what the individual really wants from the time that is left

the professional can make a difference, enabling hope – to the end of life.

It is a constant pressure not to give *false* hope; therefore keep it:

- accurate
- real
- honest

for the patient, family and yourself. Assisting the patient and family to find hope is rewarding. It is also human and that is what the caring professional is all about.

> *Acknowledging that hope is not the same as a promise means we have nothing to fear in encouraging it.*[11]

## Conclusion

People with advancing disease confront the dilemma of a shortened life and face issues of existentialism. We have a prime role in offering opportunities to patients and families for open exchange and disclosure of concerns, respecting their right to choose not to disclose.

Helping the individual to identify something positive in their life, such as close family relationships, visits from grandchildren, the love of a special person, may help to promote coping and renew hope.[15] A healing relationship between the health professional and the patient can occur when hope is mobilised.[16] We have a powerful influence on how patients respond to their illness; both in *what* we say and by *how* we say it.

The uniqueness of each human being means that coping style is individual and should be supported and respected as their method of getting through their illness.

Often, there is little to offer but ourselves, and our often unspoken understanding that we have no answers to suffering and pain. Providing comfort, attentive and thoughtful listening to the person and their family, without the offer of immediate solutions, is frequently all that we have to give – and all that is needed.

> *... Find your peace and find your place in this world*
> *Smile even when it hurts*
> *Complete your life's plan*
> *See the beauty around you, it's plentiful*
> *You'll find it in the smallest things*
> *and always remember, you are loved.*[17]

# References

1   Anderson KN, Anderson LE, Glanze WD, editors. *Mosby's Medical, Nursing and Allied Health Dictionary*, 5th edition. London: Mosby; 1998.
2   Greer S, Morris T, Pettingale KW *et al.* Psychological responses to breast cancer and 15 year outcome. *The Lancet.* 1990; **335**(i): 49–50.
3   Payne S. Coping with palliative chemotherapy. *Journal of Advanced Nursing.* 1990; **15**: 652–658.
4   Copp G, Field D. Open awareness and dying: the use of denial and acceptance as coping strategies by hospice patients. *Nursing Times Research.* 2002; **7**(2): 118–127.
5   Copp G. *Facing Impending Death: experiences of patients and their nurses.* London: Nursing Times Books; 1999.
6   Field D, Copp G. Communication and awareness about dying in the 1990s. *Palliative Medicine.* 1999; **13**: 459–468.
7   Russell GC. The role of denial in clinical practice. *Journal of Advanced Nursing.* 1999; **18**: 938–940.
8   Weisman AD. *On Dying and Denying: a psychiatric study of terminality.* New York: Behavioural Publications Inc; 1999.
9   Johnston G, Abraham C. Managing awareness: negotiating and coping with a terminal prognosis. *International Journal of Palliative Nursing.* 2000; **16**(10): 485–494.
10  Mahon SM, Cella DF, Donovan MI. Psychological adjustment to recurrent cancer. *Oncology Nursing Forum.* **17**(3): 47–52.
11  Penson J. A hope is not a promise: fostering hope within palliative care. *International Journal of Palliative Nursing.* 2000; **6**(2): 94–98.
12  Herth K. Fostering hope in terminally ill people. *Journal of Advanced Nursing.* 1990; **15**(11): 1250–1259.
13  Current Learning in Palliative Care (CLIP), 15-minute worksheet. Psychological needs: 1. Fostering hope. In: Regnard C, Kindlen M, Jackson J *et al.*, editors. *Helping the Patient with Advanced Disease: a workbook.* Oxford: Radcliffe Medical Press; 2004.
14  Buckley J, Herth K. Fostering hope in terminally ill patients. *Nursing Standard.* 2004; **19**(10): 33–41.
15  Mahon SM, Casperson DM. Exploring the psychosocial meaning of recurrent cancer: a descriptive study. *Cancer Nursing.* 1997; **20**(3): 178–186.
16  Benner P. *From Novice to Expert: excellence and power in clinical nursing practice.* California: Addison-Wesley; 1984.
17  Tremblay Cipak B. *We Are So Much Loved.* Posted at www.poetry.com; 2004.

# To learn more

• Buckley J, Herth K. Fostering hope in terminally ill patients. *Nursing Standard.* 2004; **19**(10): 33–41.
• Groopman J. *The Anatomy of Hope.* London: Simon and Schuster; 2004.
• Penson J. A hope is not a promise: fostering hope within palliative care. *International Journal of Palliative Nursing.* 2000; **6**(2): 94–98.

# Complementary chapters

*See also Stepping into Palliative Care 1: relationships and responses*

- Chapter 3: The cancer journey
- Chapter 4: The experience of illness
- Chapter 5: The psychological impact of serious illness
- Chapter 7: The therapeutic relationship

*See also Stepping into Palliative Care 2: care and practice*

- Chapter 1: Assessment in palliative care
- Chapter 11: Breaking bad news
- Chapter 12: Hearing the pain of the carer
- Chapter 13: Spirituality and palliative care

# The therapeutic relationship

*Carol Kirby*

> *For we must record love's mystery without claptrap,*
> *Snatch out of time the passionate transitory ...*[1]

## Introduction: *opening to possibility*

Therapeutic relationship is in and of itself an expression of the shared humanity at the centre of caring practice. It is primarily dialogical – a *coming-to-know* that is essentially an intellectual, emotional and existential transformation of each other's perceptions, in a context of spiritual authenticity and connection. Dialogue is the therapeutic tool through which we gain an understanding of what the person is going through and the specific meaning that the experience of illness has for them. Through dialogue, the patient's voice is heard and understood. They depend upon being heard. We respond compassionately and responsibly. In dialogue, the inner and outer world of the patient is connected and communicated to create mutual understanding.

An ethic of care, grounded in a convergence of love and 'rebellion',[2] is the emancipatory context within which therapeutic relationship achieves its goals. Within this context, an understanding of oneself as a thinker, doer and person of care, with ties that bind one to another, is potentiated. Rebellion, in the context of therapeutic relationship, reveals an impassioned concern for the dignity of each person and for the transformative action that rejects injustice and oppression while affirming human dignity, connection and concern.

The source of therapeutic relationship is the spirit of love, which opens from an innermost depth of existence to create and sustain healing. Rooted in possibility and hope it provides shelter until healing unfolds: often in the presence of fragmentation and loss. The intrinsic motivation of a caring therapeutic relation is the alleviation of suffering and the creation of liberating possibilities for another.

Caring, *caritas,* is the human mode of being: the giving of love that is a response to the call to be human. The word 'therapy' derives from the Greek word *therapeia*, which means 'care': *therapeutikos* refers to the person who provides care for another. The word 'relationship' derives from the Latin word *relatus*, denoting 'connection'. The caring connection is one of deep personal and interpersonal relation: an emotional, cognitive and spiritual interconnection. A therapeutic circle connects and responds to the existential, spiritual and physical needs of the patient. Life-affirming skilled interventions take place within negotiated-partnership practices. A competent, caring synthesis of knowledge, skill and feeling *for* and *with* the patient emerges to ensure that a sanctuary of love, trust and belonging is established. Inclusivity is primary: the patient is assured of always being involved. By including family and caring community within the caring circle, the person is understood holistically in their existential personhood and life-world, consequentially never as an object of care.

Desmond Tutu[3] captured the spirit of therapeutic relationship when he spoke of *ubuntu* – the generosity, hospitality and compassion of human being that is caught up and inextricably bound together in a humanity open to and affirming of others: humanity diminished when others are diminished.

---

**Reflective exercise 7.1**
**Time: 20 minutes**

Reflect upon Desmond Tutu's depiction of *ubuntu*.

- Consider how it relates to your experience as one caring for another.
- Speak with someone to share your experience and wisdom.

---

## Ethical encounter: *caring-healing praxis*

*Love is anything but sentimental.*
*In fact, it is the most real and creative form of human presence ...*[4]

The ethical foundation of therapeutic relationship is grounded in a sincere respect for the dignity of human life, for life's personal meaning, affirmation, significance and continual possibility. Beginning in human obligation and responsibility, in being-for-the-sake-of another, it is realised through informed and skilled compassionate caring practice. Originating in a network of interdependence, in a unity of reciprocal relationship, we come to know and to express our humanity.

The meaning we find in life is not found in individual freedom but within concerned ethical relation to one another. Emmanuel Levinas,[5] a pre-eminent continental philosopher, in his ethic of encounter speaks of the 'other's' call upon the 'I that I am', shattering indifference. The possibility invoked by the 'one-for-the-other' is a living fundamental obligation. It initiates ethical interaction. Compellingly, with respect to each person's relationship to one another, Knud Løgstrup,[6] the Danish philosopher and theologian, speaks of the primacy of 'the ethical demand'. He believes that we can take care of and help a person to the best of our ability or be indifferent to the other, ignoring or destroying a possibility to help. Whatever one's decision, whether it is to help or not, we remain demanded to do what we believe is best for the other. The other person in the situation does not make this ethical demand upon us. It is prior to and a precondition to all that we may think and consequentially do. Importantly, with respect to therapeutic relationship, it is not that I respond to the 'other' in the hope that they will likewise respond to me. I do what I do inherently as 'one-for-the-other'.

Løgstrup[6] proclaims with conviction that 'we do indeed constitute another's world and destiny'. He has said also that there are many reasons why people usually ignore this fact. Significantly, ignoring the call of the 'other' cannot be an option open within therapeutic relation. The call of another is all-important. Indispensable also is awareness that by what we do or say in relationship with another, we actually determine that person's joy or pain in living, their sincerity and serenity.

Løgstrup's[6] metaphor of '*holding another person's life in one's hand*' revealingly and powerfully depicts our ethical responsibility within caring relation. The essential is that we respond responsibly; that we do so in such a way that we do not rob any person of their independence, responsibility or human dignity.

The need for ethical commitment to uphold human dignity is convincingly made by Kay Toombs[7] when, in speaking of living and dying with dignity, she reflects upon lived experience and declares that dignity is equated with self-worth. To be treated with dignity she believes '*is to be treated with respect, to be considered worthy of the regard of others. To lose one's dignity is to feel that one's value as a person is irreparably diminished*'. An important barrier to retaining dignity in debilitating illness she asserts '*is the cultural emphasis on ''doing'' as opposed to ''being'''*. People, she has said, '*find it hard to accept that there are certain givens, inherent limitations that may derail even the most carefully constructed life plan*'. '*Recognising the difference between being and doing can be an important step in preserving self worth,*' she has poignantly declared, stating that '*if you can demonstrate to me that my illness does not degrade my worth as a person, that it is not beneath your dignity to care for me, you affirm me in a powerful manner*'. In Kay's words, all that is important has been said.

Viktor Frankl's[8] deeply humanising story of survival in Auschwitz and differing concentration camps – *Man's Search for Meaning* – responds to Kay's profound call for attention to 'being'. He offers penetrating ethical insight into the intrinsic value of human freedom, dignity and to the search for meaning that in attainment has transformative power. He proclaims a search for meaning to be the primary motivation in life: meaning, unique and specific in that it must and can only be fulfilled by each person alone and only by so doing can it achieve significance. In affirming the wisdom of Nietzsche's conviction that '*he who has a why to live for can bear almost any how*' he asserts that 'in some way, suffering ceases to be suffering at the moment it finds a meaning'. It is his belief that there is meaning in each life and that '*life retains its meaning under any conditions. It remains meaningful literally up to its last moments, up to one's last breath*'. Unavoidable suffering can have meaning if it changes one for the better, he avows.

Deborah Hutton,[9] a former health editor of *Vogue* magazine, wrote in her article 'I'm dying, but you can help me' that:

> to be ill is something we don't know how to do anymore ... and I was as bad as anyone. I took such pride in being well, superlatively well. Looking after ourselves, being well has become talismanic.

In like tone, Kay Toombs[7] (earlier spoken of), reflecting upon her lived experience of living and dying with dignity, speaks of:

> how difficult it can be for the incurably ill to retain a sense of personal dignity in the context of prevailing cultural attitudes about such things as health, independence, physical appearance, and mortality, and in the light of the almost 'magical' confidence we have in the curative power of medicine.[7]

In listening to Deborah and Kay's words, what becomes clear is the inescapable tension and fragility in life. It becomes incumbent on those caring for people who are suffering and broken 'in' and 'by' life to do what they can to assist the person to bring the broken pieces of self together again. It will help if we can make our own woundedness a source of healing connection through acknowledging self as a 'wounded healer'.

Through such caring-healing dialogue, it will be possible to assist the person to rediscover their deep sense of worth and personal dignity. This requires a trust that will enable the person to talk frankly and openly about the impact the illness is having on their lives and future goals. The imperative is that we do not hold back but that we 'hold onto' *in* and *with* faith in human possibility. Dialogue is the link to understanding what is happening in the person's life-world. Therapeutic-use-of-self is the essential compassionate response. Within the therapeutic circle, with its reliance on the person, their family and professional community, we can remove feelings of degradation and the profound sense of powerlessness and helplessness that often accompanies loss of body control. It requires not only a moral act but also, in essence, a sacred act.

---

**Reflective exercise 7.2**
**Time: 20 minutes**

Reflect upon Kay's words that, *'if you can demonstrate to me that my illness does not degrade my worth as a person, that it is not beneath your dignity to care for me, you affirm me in a powerful manner'*, while remembering Knud Løgstrup's belief that we hold *'another person's life in our hands'*.

- Consider what is being asked of us.
- Talk to someone you feel comfortable with about your feelings, certainties and uncertainties.

---

## Awakening to Spirit: *giving voice to what we know*

*All life is circular and continually changes. It has many phases. But everything, in all their different phases, is related and we must honor that relationship by giving to each other ...*[10]

To help someone to live is the great gift of human relation. To help someone to die – inspired by the love and belonging of therapeutic relation – is an honour often beyond what human words can describe. It is quintessentially a sacred bond.

When one realises that a person whose life is ending is depending upon us to be-there for them, one's consciousness of self and personal limitation may dissipate, expanding human capacities. A path, where blades of grass can spring up through concrete, may open to lead us, through unity-in-being, to finding peace-in-being and in suffering. Cicely Saunders[11] recognised that there are possibilities in people facing death that are often a source of constant astonishment. She believed that we would see it more often if we gain the confidence to approach without hiding behind a professional mask – instead, meeting one person to another; aware of the depths of pain that somehow has its healing within. Through this discovery, she has said, *'we may find out as much about living as about dying'*. Thus, we can assert that it is within deep and personal relational practice that we can assist the person and their family to cope with anguish and suffering through coming together to affirm strength and to bring forward the courage to live a meaningful life inclusive of a dignified death.

The possibilities that Cicely Saunders spoke of as '*a source of constant astonishment*' are revealed to us through an intense depth relation capable of intense possibility – creating new insights and renewed possibility for intervention. Desmond Tutu,[3] once more, speaks movingly of the intensity to life that the discovery of a life-threatening cancer made possible for him. He had renewed recognition of much that he had taken for granted – family love and devotion, the glory of a splendid sunset, the beauty of a dew-covered rose. He responded to the disease with a greater appreciation of that which he might not see or experience again. It helped him to acknowledge his mortality and to give deep thanksgiving for the very great privilege that his engagement in the healing of his nation had brought to him and to his people. He accepted that the wounds of his people, his wounds also, had enabled him to live, in the celebrated words of Henri Nouwen,[12] profoundly as a 'wounded healer'. The interpretation and personal response to his illness is testimony as to how the meaning of illness experience can transform and enhance one's life-world. It is witness to Frankl's[8] belief that unavoidable suffering does have meaning if it changes one for the better.

Arthur Kleinman[13] believes that through examining the particular significance of each person's illness it becomes possible to break the vicious cycles that amplify distress. He has said that the interpretation of illness meanings can also contribute to the provision of more effective care and that, through those interpretations, the frustrating consequences of disability can be reduced.

> *This key clinical task may even liberate sufferers and practitioners from the oppressive iron cage imposed by a too intensely morbid preoccupation with painful bodily processes and a too technically narrow and therefore dehumanizing vision of treatment, respectively.*[13]

Kleinman is steadfast in his belief that the practitioner should be-there with the patient and family in the experiential realm of suffering.

Interpretation of the experiences and meaning of illness in respect of each person, in body–mind–spirit unity, is necessary to create a holistic connected understanding and to sustain what is often fragile hope. Individual suffering is in every way unique. Access to the suffering and loss that a person is experiencing is inalienably theirs to give. It is an arrogance, intended or not, to believe that we *know* anything of another's experience except through their telling. The necessity is to accept, unconditionally, each person's separateness: at the same time mindful that we need each other; that we live connected in our humanity. *Humanity is the place*, David Roy[14] believes, *where you will find someone who will enter into your suffering and never leave you there alone.*

Each person is living and experiencing their unfolding life and its meaning, daily finding and renewing meaning. It is not possible to confer meaning upon another person's life. What is possible and vital within therapeutic relation is the assistance of the person to find meaning in what they are going through or, in the words of Joyce Travelbee,[15] '*to find meaning in their suffering*'. The crucial is that we are present to the person as they enter the deepest dimensions of their being in search of spiritual connection and existential meaning. The obligatory is that we attempt always to understand and to help the person feel understood by going beyond the everyday way of relation to therapeutic endeavour.

The physician and writer Bert Keizer[16] believes that it hurts when essential existential questions are ignored or covered over by what is often a chase for scientific answers. It is compounded by a failure to stand by the patient in their suffering. It hurts, he has said, when faceless biochemistry is offered when one is trying to digest one's suffering religiously, metaphysically or psychologically. He believes that silly reverence for scientific questions and answers ignores the suffering that cannot be taken away. He has said that *'ignoring a person's suffering because all the attention is focused on biochemical parameters is a daily sin'*. Yet it happens all too frequently in a healthcare world often torn between caring and curing.

---

**Reflective exercise 7.3**
**Time: 15 minutes**

*'Everything that happens to each one of us has potential to deepen and transform us.'*

- Consider this statement and record your response.

---

## Stepping into the Light: *awakening-belonging*

*... and a tranquil candle burns ...*

Therapeutic relationship began a discovery of the need that each person had for the 'other' – that each deeply mattered to one another. It recognised that the all-important was a capacity to invest someone with hope; to invoke healing power from within the person in an engagement of patient and family supported within a skilled, compassionate, caring community. The therapeutic circle provided the vital context to effect caring-healing practice.

We have come to recognise that we are each at once actual and potential and that the in-between is the *possible* – the ethical space where possibility and potential are realised. We journeyed into the world held onto with caring hands: we journey out of the world held closer with caring hands and heart. Love and human care light the way.

Caring-healing practice required the convergence of clinical competence with compassionate understanding. It recognised that the care-requiring and care-giving existential voices are inextricably interwoven within vital ethical interaction. In the technologised world of healthcare, the caring voice resonates humanity; the human heart opens and responds in caring presence within the ethical space.

Ethical conviction and connection is achieved within an ethic of care characterised in the inextricably interwoven virtues of:

- *authentic being* – realising potential, renewing being
- *conscience* – consciousness, engagement in moral activity, awareness creation
- *commitment* – advocate with, 'with' when the other has no choice but to be-there
- *presence* – being-with, confirmation of the other, constancy and immediacy of relationship
- *compassion* – interdependence, feeling *for* and *with*, concern of care
- *empathy* – involvement, acceptance of, understanding the way of the other
- *empowerment* – liberation, freedom to realise potential, mutual understanding and confirmation.

---

Reflective exercise 7.4
Time: 15 minutes

Reflect upon the opening words *'and a tranquil candle burns ...'*.

- Spontaneously record in written form thoughts and feelings brought to mind.

---

## Conclusion

Love is life giving, life sustaining. We live love's mystery: in relation responding. We see clearly, understand deeply. It is the essence of therapeutic caring practice.

## References

1  Kavanagh P. The hospital. In: Stack T, editor. *No Earthly Estate: God and Patrick Kavanagh – an anthology*. Blackrock, Dublin: Columba Press; 2002.
2  Camus A. *The Rebel: An essay on man in revolt*. New York: Random House; 1956.
3  Tutu D. *No Future Without Forgiveness*. London: Rider; 1999.
4  O'Donohue J. *Anam Ćara*. London: Bantam Press; 1997.
5  Levinas E. *On Thinking-of-the-Other Entre Nous*. London: The Athlone Press; 1998.
6  Løgstrup KE. *The Ethical Demand*. London: University of Notre Dame Press; 1997.
7  Toombs SK. Living and dying with dignity: reflections on lived experience. *Journal of Palliative Care*. 2004; **20**(3): 193–200.
8  Frankl VE. *Man's Search for Meaning*. London: Rider; 2004.
9  Hutton D. I'm dying, but you can help me. *The Sunday Times, News Review*. 2005; **10 July**: 3.
10  Brown Otter. Cited in: M Pflüg. Pimadaziwin: contemporary rituals in Odawa community. In: Irwin L, editor. *Native American Spirituality: a critical reader*. Lincoln: University of Nebraska Press; 2000.
11  Saunders C. Foreword. In: Kearney M. *Mortally Wounded – stories of soul pain, death and healing*. Dublin: Marino; 1996.
12  Nouwen H. *The Wounded Healer*. New York: Image; 1972.
13  Kleinman A. *The Illness Narratives: suffering, healing, and the human condition*. New York: Basic Books; 1998.
14  Roy DJ. Humanity: idea, image, reality. *Journal of Palliative Care*. 2004; **20**(3): 131–132.
15  Travelbee J. *Interpersonal Aspects of Nursing*, 2nd edition. Philadelphia: FA Davis Company; 1971.
16  Keizer B. Living well, dying well (1). In: Marinker M, editor. *Medicine and Humanity*. London: King's Fund; 2001.

## To learn more

- Kirby C. Commitment to care: a philosophical perspective on nursing. In: Basford L, Slevin O, editors. *Theory and Practice of Nursing: an integrated approach to caring practice*. Cheltenham: Nelson Thornes; 2003.
- Kirby C. The therapeutic relationship. In: Basford L, Slevin O, editors. *Theory and Practice of Nursing: an integrated approach to caring practice*. Cheltenham: Nelson Thornes: 2003.

# Complementary chapters

*See also Stepping into Palliative Care 1: relationships and responses*

- Chapter 1: Learning to learn in palliative care
- Chapter 3: The cancer journey
- Chapter 4: The experience of illness
- Chapter 5: The psychological impact of serious illness
- Chapter 6: Hope and coping strategies
- Chapter 16: Sexuality and palliative care

*See also Stepping into Palliative Care 2: care and practice*

- Chapter 10: Terminal restlessness
- Chapter 11: Breaking bad news
- Chapter 13: Spirituality and palliative care
- Chapter 14: Bereavement

# Chapter 8

# Gold Standards Framework: a programme for community palliative care

*Keri Thomas and Helen Meehan*

---

**Pre-reading exercise 8.1**
**Time: 20 minutes**

- Reflect on the role of primary care in your area in caring for palliative care patients.
- Reflect on the care of a patient that has gone well and the care of a patient that has not gone well. What are the learning points?

---

## Introduction

Few things in primary care are more important and more rewarding than enabling a patient to die peacefully at home. Many GPs, district nurses and others in the primary healthcare team (PHCT) feel that palliative care represents the best of all medical and nursing care, bringing together clinical, holistic and human dimensions of care. Caring for the dying and supporting patients near the last stage of life is an important and intrinsic area of their work. Primary care plays a vitally important role for patients in the last years of life. Primary care teams deliver the majority of hands-on palliative and supportive care to patients and generally do this in a sound and effective way, especially when backed by specialist palliative care support.[1] Although there are many examples of good care, sometimes care can be uncoordinated, inconsistent and reactive, leading to a variable standard of care. One means of improving the consistency and quality of care within the community is to use the Gold Standards Framework (GSF). This tried and tested framework offers PHCTs an evidence-based programme with tools and resources to help improve the organisation and planning of palliative care for their patients in the community.[2]

*The aim of the Gold Standards Framework* is to develop a practice-based system to improve the organisation and quality of care for patients in the last stages of life in the community, so that more live and die well in their preferred place of choice.

This framework is now extensively used across the UK with approximately a quarter of GP practices using GSF in some way. It has been supported by national policy in England including the National Institute for Clinical Excellence (NICE) guidance for supportive and palliative care (2004),[3] the NHS End of Life Care Programme and the Royal College of General Practitioners. It is recommended as a model of good practice for optimising delivery of good palliative care in the community (*see* Box 8.1).

---

**Box 8.1    Key components of best practice in community palliative care – Gold Standards Framework[3]**

1  Patients with needs for palliative care are identified according to agreed criteria and a management plan discussed within the multidisciplinary team.
2  These patients and their carers are regularly assessed using agreed assessment tools.
3  Anticipated needs are noted, planned for and addressed.
4  Patient and carer needs are communicated within the team and to specialist colleagues as appropriate.
5  Preferred place of care and place of death are discussed and noted, and measures taken to comply where possible.
6  Coordination of care is orchestrated by a named person in the practice team.
7  Relevant information is passed to those providing care out of hours, and anticipated drugs left in the home.
8  A protocol for care in the dying phase is followed, such as the Liverpool Care Pathway for the Dying Patient.
9  Carers are educated, enabled and supported, which includes the provision of specific information, financial advice and bereavement care.
10 Audit, reflective practice, development of practice protocols and targeted learning are encouraged as part of personal, practice and primary care organisation/NHS trust development plans.

---

GSF is not a prescriptive model but a framework that can be adapted according to local needs and resources. The GSF:

● enables teams to build on the good practice already present
● supports consistency of good coordinated care with a more patient-centred focus
● improves communication within and between teams.

However, GSF is only part of the jigsaw needed to improve end-of-life care across a whole healthcare community. Along with other developments such as:

● improved advanced care planning
● better patient and carer support
● communication skills
● care in the dying phase
● integrated care pathways (for example, Liverpool Care Pathway).

GSF can support and enable improved care along the whole patient journey and contribute an important role in end-of-life care.

GSF is a generic tool developed from primary care for primary care, initially for cancer patients, but now widely used for any patient with a life-limiting illness. The framework was piloted first in West Yorkshire and then developed into a phased programme of spread supported by the Cancer Services Collaborative and Macmillan Cancer Support. GSF is now part of the NHS End of Life Care Programme in England. A separate Gold Standards Framework Scotland Project has been funded for 3 years. Macmillan Cancer Support also supports the use of GSF in Northern Ireland and in Wales.

## NHS End of Life Care Programme

The NHS End of Life Care Programme has been established to help:

- professionals improve the quality of care at the end of life for all patients
- enable more patients to live and die in the place of their choice.

The definition used for these patients is that they have an advanced progressive, eventually fatal illness and are in need of supportive care, as they approach the end of their lives. It includes care given in the terminal stages and for some patients may include care for several years. The programme objective is to '*offer all adult patients nearing the end of life, regardless of diagnosis, the choice and access to high quality end of life care*'.[4]

The key outcomes for the End of Life Care Programme are outlined in Box 8.2. To support these outcomes the End of Life Care Programme promotes the use of GSF as one of the quality-improvement tools.

---

Box 8.2    The NHS End of Life Care Programme anticipated outcomes

- Greater choice for patients in their place of care and place of death.
- Decrease in the number of emergency admissions for patients who have expressed a wish to die at home.
- Decrease in the number of patients transferred from a care home to district general hospital in the last week of life.
- Generalists skilled in the use of the models of care tools to improve end-of-life care.

---

Self-assessment exercise 8.1
Time: 15 minutes

1  In which setting would you expect to find implementation of GSF?
2  What is the aim of GSF and how would you summarise it?
3  Name a national policy document that supports implementation of GSF.

## Context of palliative care in the community

Most patients when asked say they would prefer to remain at home, and to die there, if possible, if they and their carers are supported. As a second choice, many choose hospice care. Wherever someone eventually dies, most time will be spent at home in the last year of life, so providing the best home care for the final stage of life will always be important.

- Supportive and palliative care towards the end of life will be increasingly needed in future with predicted demographic changes – the ageing population is living longer with serious illness, with fewer people available to care for them.[5]
- Overall, most palliative care is provided by generalists and demand outstrips supply of specialist support. Optimising primary and specialist services to enable full and complementary provision will maximise benefits for patients.[1]
- The majority would prefer to die at home (with hospice as second choice), but only about a quarter die there, yet over half die in hospitals, despite a small minority choosing this. For many the place of death is by default rather than by choice, due to lack of planning or service provision, problems with symptom control or carer support.[6,7]
- Hospital death is more likely for the poor, elderly, women, those with a long illness, etc. Government policy aims to reduce inappropriate hospital usage. So, enabling more dying people to remain at home is increasingly important.[8]

Therefore, there is a drive towards providing more effective and reliable community-based care. This would include maximising the generalist provision in primary care, intermediate care, hospice and hospice-at-home services, care homes, social services, etc.

---

**Self-assessment exercise 8.2**
**Time: 5 minutes**

1 Where currently do the patients spend the majority of their last year of life?
2 Why will there be an increasing need for supportive and palliative care in the future?

---

## Underlying assumption of GSF

GSF was developed as a means to improve the *in-hours* care for patients nearing the end of life to prevent *out-of-hours* crises. The underlying processes include:

- these patients being *identified*
- their needs being *assessed*
- the primary care team then proactively *planning* care.

Throughout these processes *communication* is of paramount importance, not only within the primary care team and with patients and their carers, but also with those involved with providing care and support along the patient journey. This could include hospital teams, specialist palliative care, social services, 'out-of-hours' providers, care homes, etc. GSF centres on the needs of patients and their families and encourages interprofessional primary care teams to work together.

## What will GSF improve?

*GSF is magic! It is MUCH more than it first appears – it is like a key that unlocks the creativity of people, and releases the potential for a new way of working for the whole team. It helps us do what we already want to do, but even better. Now we really do talk to each other – it has transformed the way we care for our very ill patients, and has put us back in touch with the reasons we are doing this job in the first place.* (GP and district nurse, West Midlands, 2005)

Since its development, GSF has had university-led (Warwick and Birmingham) evaluation and measurement of outcomes. From these initial and ongoing evaluations of GSF nationally there have been identified improvements for patients, carers, PHCTs and service development. Evidence shows that there is improved:

- communication – within and between teams, with patients and their families
- coordination and organisation of care by the PHCT
- proactive planning of care and communication between service providers including *out of hours*
- patient-focused care using holistic assessments
- information for patients and carers
- bereavement support
- evaluation and auditing within primary care informing development of local services
- partnership working with specialist palliative care.

Practice review and audit is an integral part of GSF, as are measures to improve consistency and dependability of care provided. Many practices and PCTs have developed ongoing GSF audit cycles to support sustainability of GSF and enable continued review of palliative care within primary care.

Information on the evaluations and research articles can be found on the GSF website: www.goldstandardsframework.nhs.uk.

## GSF in practice

GSF is a simple common-sense approach to formalising best practice, so that good care becomes standard for all patients every time. GPs, district nurses and practice teams find it affirms good practice, standardises quality palliative care activities and improves consistency of care.

The framework includes strategies, tasks and enabling tools to support teams in the community to improve coordination and care planning for patients with a life-limiting illness. GSF can be summarised into three processes, five goals and seven standards, as outlined in Box 8.3.

---

**Box 8.3    The Gold Standards Framework 1, 3, 5, 7 summary**

1    **Aim** – one chance to aim for the best for all – one 'gold standard' to aspire to for *all* patients nearing the end of life, whatever the diagnosis, stage or setting.

3    **Central processes of GSF** – all involving improved communication, are to:

   • identify patients in need of palliative/supportive care towards the end of life
   • assess their needs, symptoms, preferences and any issues important to them
   • plan care around patients' needs and preferences and enable these to be fulfilled, in particular allow patients to live and die where they choose.

5    **Main goals** of GSF are to provide high quality care for people in the final months of life in the community:

   • patients are as symptom controlled as possible
   • place of care – patients are enabled to live well and die well in their preferred place of choice
   • security and support – better advanced care planning, information, less fear, fewer crises/admissions to hospital
   • carers are supported, informed, enabled and empowered
   • staff confidence, communication and co-working are improved.

7    **Gold standards** of community palliative care or the 7 Cs:

   • C1 Communication
   • C2 Coordination
   • C3 Control of symptoms
   • C4 Continuity including out of hours
   • C5 Continued learning
   • C6 Carer support
   • C7 Care in the dying phase.

---

# The 7 Cs or standards to GSF in practice

## *C1 Communication*

Practices maintain a supportive care register (paper or electronic) to record, plan and monitor patient care, and as a tool to discuss at regular PHCT meetings.

The aims of the meetings are to improve:

• the flow of communication
• advanced care planning and proactive care
• measurement and audit, to clarify areas for future improvement at patient, practice, PCT (primary care trust) and network level.

Communication and sharing of information using Advanced Care Planning tools are recommended, to ensure that the wishes of the patient are discussed and recorded. The Advanced Care Plan should include information on preferred place of care, 'Do Not Resuscitate' issues, proxy, organ donation, etc.

## C2 Coordination

Each PHCT has a nominated coordinator for palliative care (e.g. district nurse) to ensure good organisation and coordination of care in a practice by overseeing the process:

- maintaining a register of problems/concerns, summary care plans, symptom sheets, handover forms, audit data, etc.
- organising the PHCT meetings for discussion, planning, case analysis, education, etc.
- using tools for symptom assessment.

## C3 Control of symptoms

Each patient has their symptoms, problems and concerns (physical, psychological, social, practical and spiritual) assessed, recorded, discussed and acted upon, according to an agreed process. The focus is more on the patient agenda. The use of Symptom Control Assessment tools, e.g. for pain assessment, are recommended, as well as Advanced Care Planning tools as described in C1 Communication. (For examples of assessment tools *see* GSF website.)

## C4 Continuity

Systems and protocols should be developed to ensure continuity of care delivered by interprofessional teams and out-of-hours providers. Practices will transfer information to the out-of-hours service for palliative care patients, e.g. using a handover form and out-of-hours protocol.

This builds in anticipatory care to reduce crises and inappropriate admissions. Information should also be passed on to other relevant services, e.g. hospice/ oncology department (using patient-held record and medication cards). Record and minimise the number of professionals involved, e.g. note the lead GP, lead district nurse and deputy for each patient.

## C5 Continued learning

The primary care team will continue interprofessional learning focused on real clinical problems, consistent with adult learning principles. The PHCT will be committed to continued learning of skills and information relevant to patients seen: 'learn as you go'.

Using practice-based or external teaching, lectures, videos, significant event analysis (SEA) or other tools, the practice and personal development plans and audits/appraisals are implemented. The practice develops a learning and reference resource.

Learning is clinical, organisational/strategic and also attitude/approach, e.g. communication skills in holding difficult conversations related to planning and preference of care.

## C6 Carer support

This approach encourages practices to work in partnerships with carers and also to consider their needs, including the following:

- *Emotional support* – carers are supported, listened to, kept informed and encouraged to play as full a role in the patient's care as they and the patient wish. They are regarded as an integral part of the caring team.
- *Practical support* – practical hands-on support is supplied where possible, e.g. night sitter, respite care, day hospice, equipment, etc.
- *Bereavement support* – practices plan support, e.g. developing a practice bereavement protocol, visits, notes tagged, others informed as appropriate.
- *Staff support* – is inbuilt and nurtured leading to better teamwork and job satisfaction.

## C7 Care of the dying

Patients in the last days of life (terminal phase) are cared for appropriately, e.g. by using the minimum protocol or following the Liverpool Care Pathway.

This includes stopping non-essential interventions and drugs, considering comfort measures, psychological and religious/spiritual support, bereavement planning, communication and care after death being assessed and recorded.

---

**Self-assessment exercise 8.3**
**Time: 15 minutes**

1 What is a supportive care register in a GSF practice?
2 What are the 7Cs of GSF?
3 What is an advanced care plan?

---

# How to implement GSF

Although individual practices can undertake GSF separately, it is much stronger and more sustainable if a group of practices adopt the framework together, and collectively change service provision in their area or PCT. They can then fully integrate GSF into their palliative care protocols, assessment tools, guidelines, education, clinical governance agenda, etc.

The GSF Programme in England, funded by NHS End of Life Care Programme, has largely functioned on a 'cascade' principle (*see* Figure 8.1) of enabling and supporting local people to facilitate GSF in their own area, giving it local flavour, relevance and ownership. GSF has been adopted and adapted in rural and urban areas alike, among varying circumstances and degrees of specialist palliative care provision, but the basic principles can be modified to best suit each area, with shared learning via this national momentum.

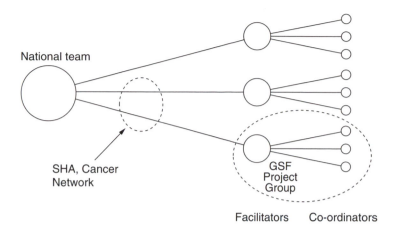

**Figure 8.1**  National GSF cascade support programme.

The GSF facilitator supports the GSF practices, organises local GSF meetings, registration of practices and collection of GSF audit questionnaires to send to the national GSF team. The national GSF team then supports the PCT facilitators through workshops, an advice line, newsletters and website resources.

It is easiest to take GSF in stages. Box 8.4 shows the levels of GSF implementation as the different seven standards are introduced within a practice. It is also possible for PCTs and strategic health authorities to use the levels of implementation to audit adoption of GSF across an area.

---

**Box 8.4  GSF levels of implementation**

**Level 1:** C1 and C2

- Set up the register.
- Organise the PHCT meetings.
- Clarify the role of the nominated coordinator.

**Level 2:** C3, C4 and C5

- Add in better assessment of symptoms and clinical management.
- Improve out-of-hours continuity with handover forms, etc.
- Build in targeted learning, e.g. invite the Macmillan CNS (clinical nurse specialist)/specialist palliative care nurses to discuss cases with you.
- Measure continuously and reflect on developments using SEA when appropriate.

**Level 3:** C6 and C7

- Add improved information for carers (e.g. using home packs, carers' information pack, local information on services).
- Better support for carers.

- When reaching the terminal stages, examine your agreed protocol for the last days of life and use suggestions made.

**Level 4**: Sustain, embed, extend

- Reflect back analysis of data to local commissioners to improve services, e.g. main causes of inappropriate admissions, deficiencies in local services.
- Develop your own practice protocol with local details, allocated personnel, etc.
- Collaborate with your facilitator, primary care organisation/network to commission better services for your patients.
- Include non-cancer patients in supportive care (SC) register if not already included.
- Discuss as a team any new ideas and suggestions on how you will routinely provide supportive care for your seriously ill or dying patients.

The first level may take about 2–3 months to establish, but all can be achieved within 12 months. A few practice teams remain at level 1, with just the register and a regular meeting, but most benefit is gained when teams develop and integrate GSF more deeply into levels 2, 3 and 4.

## GSF and proactive patient care?

The benefits of implementing GSF are shown in Table 8.1, through a patient journey before use of GSF compared to that of a patient journey after implementation of GSF. It demonstrates how GSF can enable primary care teams to work more proactively and how it can improve the patient's experience of care.

Table 8.1   Reactive (pre-GSF) and proactive patient journey (post-GSF)

| Patient Mr B: reactive patient journey | Patient Mrs W: proactive patient journey |
| --- | --- |
| • GP and DN (district nurse) ad hoc arrangements – no preferred place of death discussed or anticipated.<br>• Problems with symptom control – high anxiety.<br>• Crisis call *out of hours* – no plan or drugs available in the home.<br>• Admitted to hospital.<br>• Dies in hospital.<br>• Carer given minimal support in grief.<br>• No reflection by PHCT team on care given.<br>• Inappropriate use of hospital bed? | • On SC register – discussed at PHCT meeting (C1).<br>• DS1500 and info given to patient and carer (home pack) (C1, C6).<br>• Regular support, visits, phone calls – proactive (C1, C2).<br>• Assessment of symptoms, partnership with specialist palliative care (SPC) – customised care to patient and carer needs (C3).<br>• Carer assessed including psychosocial needs (C3, C6).<br>• Preferred place of care noted and organised (C1, C2).<br>• Handover form issued – care plan and drugs issued for home (C4).<br>• End-of-life pathway/Liverpool Care Pathway (LCP)/minimum protocol used (C7).<br>• Patient dies in preferred place – bereavement support. Staff reflect –SEA, audit gaps, improve care, learn (C5, C6). |

## Palliative care specialists and GSF

Palliative care specialists, including doctors, nurses and hospice staff, play a key role in the support and delivery of GSF in an area, and it is vital to involve them from the start. Their central role in delivering and improving community palliative care services will also be greatly enhanced by their support for primary care teams in using GSF. It will only be by real collaboration of generalists and specialists that effective improvements in community palliative care can be made.

In many areas the implementation of GSF has affirmed the role of specialist palliative care and enabled greater partnership with primary care teams. Some examples of dovetailing specialist palliative care services with primary care through GSF have included:

- continued affirmation of the value and role of the generalist in palliative care and care of the dying
- practices having an allocated named palliative care clinical nurse specialist (CNS) to support them with symptom control advice, care planning, attending PHCT meetings when palliative care patients are discussed
- specialist palliative care support with development of guidelines and local protocols, e.g. clinical symptom management, formularies, out-of-hours protocols
- facilitation of Significant Event Analysis or Traffic-Light sessions with primary care teams, looking at what was good, what was not so good and ideas for further improvement
- support with practice-based educational sessions on palliative care
- developing agreed palliative care assessment tools to be used locally.

## Non-cancer diagnosis and GSF

GSF is fully adaptable for patients with a non-cancer diagnosis in need of end-of-life care. Through national evaluation it is known that the majority of practices use the framework for non-cancer within 6 months of implementing GSF. However, there is a need to develop criteria for including non-cancer patients in the supportive care register (*see* the GSF website for current information). This is in line with the objectives of the NHS End of Life Care Programme to '*offer all adult patients nearing the end of life, regardless of diagnosis, the choice and access to high quality end of life care*'.

## Education and GSF

Best patient care will only occur when there is a combination of three areas:

- *head* – clinical expertise – *head* knowledge
- *hands* – organisational processes
- *heart* – patient focus.

So, best palliative care will not occur just by educating healthcare staff, but by also changing systems of practice. Likewise GSF will not work well unless complemented by an increasing knowledge base, *learn-as-you-go* thinking and access to specialist support. So education and continued learning is intrinsic to GSF as one of the seven key standards.

To enable best care we recognise the need for interprofessional learning, focusing on real clinical problems, consistent with adult learning principles. GSF encourages practice-based learning through the use of videos, reflective practice, personal development plans, practice review meetings, specialist palliative care teaching and support. Education for carers is also intrinsic in continued learning and means of improving carers' understanding and expectations are also encouraged.

## Care homes and GSF

Patients in care homes in the community (nursing or residential homes) come under the medical care of GPs and PHCTs. Many practices included patients from care homes on their GSF supportive care registers, but felt that a modified version of GSF could be used in care homes themselves.

GSF for care homes (GSFCH) was seen therefore as a simple extension of the care provided by the GP/primary care team in the community, underpinned with the same basic principles and criteria. However, there are many particular challenges in care-home palliative care provision, such as the private/NHS care partnerships, multiple co-morbidities, concomitant mental incapacity, staff turnover and cultural differences. Twenty per cent of the population die in care homes. Therefore, optimising care in this area is a vital part of improving end-of-life care for all.

The GSF national team is undertaking an action research study implementing and evaluating GSF within the care homes setting. A phase 1 report is available on the website. Phase 2 has 100 care homes nationally implementing GSFCH and a 'good practice guide' will be developed. Evaluation is led by a team from Birmingham University. More details on this are available from the GSF central team and the GSF website.

## Conclusion

With the post-baby-boom demographic timebomb ahead of us, the most significant challenge we face in service provision is to enable more people to live well and die well in the place and in the manner of their choosing. Practically speaking, this means raising the quality and reliability of services provided by all, and to reduce crises and unneeded hospital admissions. So within primary care there is a pressing need for active anticipatory management, coordination and care planning to enable more patients to live out their days well and to die in the place of their choosing. GSF has been developed to support teams working in primary care to deliver this proactive, coordinated care for their patients. GSF helps to improve the reliability of home care by mainstreaming the ideals of palliative care into standard practice and is a key part of improving end-of-life care for everyone.

> *Mission impossible? Palliative care at home embraces what is most noble in medicine: sometimes curing, always relieving, supporting right to the end.*[9]

# References

1   Mitchell G. How well do general practitioners deliver palliative care? A systematic review. *Palliative Medicine.* 2002; **16**: 457–464.
2   Thomas K. *Caring for the Dying at Home: companions on the journey.* Oxford: Radcliffe Medical Press; 2003.
3   National Institute for Clinical Excellence. *Improving Supportive and Palliative Care for Adults with Cancer.* London: NICE; 2004.
4   www.endoflifecare.nhs.uk.
5   World Health Organization (WHO). *Better Palliative Care for Older People.* Milan, Italy: WHO; 2004.
6   Thorpe G. Enabling more dying people to remain at home. *BMJ.* 1993; **307**: 915–918.
7   Thomas C, Morris SM, Clark D. Place of death: preferences among cancer patients and their carers. *Social Science and Medicine.* 2004; **58**: 2431–2444.
8   Higginson IJ, Astin P, Dolan S. Where do cancer patients die? Ten year trend in the place of death of cancer patients in England. *Palliative Medicine.* 1998; **12**: 353–363.
9   Gomas JM. Palliative care at home: reality or mission impossible? *Palliative Medicine.* 1993; **7**: 45–59.

# To learn more

- For more information on the NHS End of Life Care Programme tools visit: www.endoflifecare.nhs.uk.
- To learn more about GSF and contact the GSF Central Team visit: www.goldstandardsframework.nhs.uk.

# Complementary chapters

*See also Stepping into Palliative Care 1: relationships and responses*

- Chapter 1: Learning to learn in palliative care
- Chapter 2: What is palliative care?
- Chapter 3: The cancer journey
- Chapter 4: The experience of illness
- Chapter 9: Integrated care pathways
- Chapter 11: The value of teamwork
- Chapter 13: Communication: the essence of good practice, management and leadership

*See also Stepping into Palliative Care 2: care and practice*

- Chapter 1: Assessment in palliative care
- Chapter 9: The last few days of life
- Chapter 10: Terminal restlessness
- Chapter 13: Spirituality and palliative care
- Chapter 14: Bereavement
- Chapter 16: The special needs of the neurological patient

# Integrated care pathways

*John E Ellershaw*

## Introduction

When a patient presents with a problem (e.g. pain), the healthcare professional involved responds by assessing the symptom and suggesting the most appropriate intervention (e.g. analgesics). This in itself appears to be a routine process, but what of the outcome of the intervention? How do we measure whether the treatment prescribed has actually helped? What do we do if it has not?

---

**Self-assessment exercise 9.1**
**Time: 1 hour**

Choose a specific symptom, e.g. pain, and review your assessment and the success of your intervention regarding:

1  an individual patient
2  all patients over the past month.

---

This set of questions begins to challenge how we measure the outcomes of care. Increasingly, we are being asked to demonstrate clinical effectiveness.[1,2] This is not only about the process of delivery of care, but also – importantly – about the outcomes of care.

Within palliative care, the philosophy of care is patient centred and acknowledges the importance of dealing not only with the physical aspects but also with the psychosocial and spiritual dimensions of care.

If then we are to measure outcomes of care, is this not too complex a task to undertake? A number of tools have been developed that examine some or all of the domains of care, and others attempt to measure the patient's 'quality of life'.[3] Many of these tools are additional to the already considerable workload of healthcare professionals, and few of them have been incorporated successfully into everyday practice. Does this therefore suggest that palliative care is special and we are trying to measure unmeasurable outcomes?

This is one conclusion that we may draw. However, there are problems associated with it. First, it invites criticism that if we cannot demonstrate the outcomes of our care, then we are unable to highlight areas of effective practice and other areas that could improve patient care with further education, resources and/or research. Second, if funding of services is directed to areas of clinical effectiveness, as demonstrated by outcome measures, then palliative care might find itself well down the priority list.

Therefore, there are good reasons to suggest that measuring outcomes in palliative care is worthwhile. What role then, if any, do integrated care pathways (ICPs) have in meeting this need?

## What is an ICP?

ICPs have been developed and established in the North American healthcare system, and more recently have been adopted in the UK.[4,5] They are used in a wide range of conditions outside palliative care including chest pain, breast disease and leg ulcers.[6,7] ICPs provide guidelines and appropriate supporting documentation is included in the pathway for reference. The ICP is central to the patient's care, and is completed by all healthcare professionals involved with the patient. Thus it *replaces all other documentation.*

## How are ICPs initiated?

To undertake the development of an ICP for a whole service (e.g. palliative care) is an ambitious goal.[8] It is advisable to start by identifying an episode or part of patient care that can be developed into an ICP. Following the implementation of an ICP for part of a service, it then becomes easier to develop additional ICPs that link together. For example, in palliative care an ICP for the dying patient has been developed (the Liverpool Care of the Dying Pathway [LCP] )[9,10] to encompass the last days/hours of life. Following successful implementation of the ICP of the dying patient, it is then possible to develop an ICP for initial assessment of palliative care patients and their ongoing review.

Once a discrete part of a service has been identified for ICP development, all professionals involved in care of the patient during that episode must meet to identify the goals of care. It is essential that all disciplines are involved at this stage of development and have ownership; otherwise implementation will be far more difficult. When developing an ICP for the dying patient, this would include nurses and doctors as the core team, but might include chaplains, social workers, occupational therapists and physiotherapists, depending on local circumstances.

## How to write an ICP

It is important that an ICP is locally owned. Although there is value in reviewing other care pathways that have been developed, adaptation and further development will be necessary to render them appropriate for local use. The first step is to identify achievable goals, referred to as *'outcomes of care'*. This is done by retrospective review of case-notes and by discussion within the team to identify the key outcomes of care.

In care of the dying these *'outcomes of care'* can be categorised into the following three phases of care:

1 initial assessment and care, when the patient is identified as being in the dying phase (i.e. the healthcare workers have agreed that the patient is dying and has only hours or days to live)
2 ongoing care of the dying patient
3 care of relatives after death.

---

**Self-assessment exercise 9.2**
**Time: 1 hour**

Consider the last three palliative care patients for whom you have provided care, and identify the key outcomes of care for the first phase (i.e. when the patient was identified as dying).

---

An example of outcomes of care for this phase is given in Box 9.1.

---

**Box 9.1    Initial assessment – outcomes of care**

**Comfort measures:**
*Goal 1*: Current medication assessed and non-essentials discontinued.
*Goal 2*: PRN subcutaneous medication written up as per protocol (pain, agitation, respiratory tract secretions).
*Goal 3*: Discontinue inappropriate interventions (blood tests, antibiotics).

**Psychological insight:**
*Goal 4*: Insight into condition identified for patient.
*Goal 5*: Insight into condition identified for carer (carer understands the patient is dying).

**Religious support:**
*Goal 6*: Religious needs identified/discussed with patient/carer.

**Communication:**
*Goal 7*: Plan of care explained and discussed with patient/family/other.
*Goal 8*: Family/others express understanding of plan of care.

*Adapted from the Liverpool Care Pathway for the Dying Patient.*

---

When identifying key outcomes of care, national/local guidelines and research-based evidence should be utilised and incorporated whenever possible. Having identified the key outcomes of care, *'prompts'* that enable the outcome to be 'achieved' or 'not achieved' (e.g. a variance) are added beneath each goal. Box 9.2 gives an example of an outcome (goal 2) and supporting prompts in the initial assessment section of the LCP.

---

**Box 9.2    Example of goal 2 from initial assessment section in the ICP for the dying patient**

**Goal:** PRN subcutaneous medication written up from list below. Yes ☐    No ☐
    *Pain*:                      analgesia.                Yes ☐    No ☐
    *Agitation*:             sedative.                 Yes ☐    No ☐
    *Respiratory tract secretions*:  anticholinergic.     Yes ☐    No ☐

*Adapted from the Liverpool Care Pathway for the Dying Patient.*

This initial writing of an ICP takes at least three meetings. It is advisable to have a facilitator with some knowledge of pathway development in order to complete the development phase as effectively as possible. To increase ownership of the final document, it is important to circulate the draft document as widely as possible among the healthcare professionals who are ultimately going to use it for comment. It is helpful to amend the ICP following consultation, but there is no such thing as a perfect or definitive ICP. An important feature of using the ICP is that it is constantly undergoing scrutiny and changing to adapt to local need and wider developments.

## Implementing an ICP

Figure 9.1 shows the developmental steps from a case-oriented culture to a culture of excellence in clinical practice. Too often organisations leap from step 1 straight to using complex outcome measures (step 5). This is perhaps one of the reasons why so few outcome measures have been incorporated into palliative care practice. By adopting a culture that moves towards outcome-based practice (e.g. by the development of ICPs), more complex outcome measures can then be incorporated into the ICP. For example, we may decide to have as a goal for initial assessment in palliative care the fact that the patient is *'pain free'*.

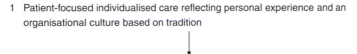

1  Patient-focused individualised care reflecting personal experience and an organisational culture based on tradition

2  Recognition that outcomes of care should influence practice

3  Shift in the culture of organisation to recognise the value of outcome-based practice

4  Introduction of outcome-based practice with feedback of outcomes to staff that identify areas of high achievement and also areas where education or additional resources may further improve care

5  Incorporation of externally developed measures and increasing attention to evidence-based practice

6  Organisation has a fully developed evidence-based practice with measurable outcomes and a culture which can respond appropriately to new developments within the field of expertise

7  Patient-focused individualised care reflecting evidence-based practice and an organisational culture based on continuous improvement

**Figure 9.1**   Development steps towards outcome-based practice.

Initially we can record a basic measurement (e.g. whether pain is present or absent). However, it may then be possible to incorporate more complex measurements (e.g. a Visual Analogue Scale – VAS) into our assessment. Future analysis will then give a more accurate reflection of the patient's pain control and how it changes over time.

The time taken to change the culture of an organisation may range from months to years, and must not be underestimated if the implementation of the ICP is to be effective.

## Associated guidelines

In the writing of the ICP, national/local guidelines and research-based evidence should be incorporated whenever possible. It may also be considered helpful by the team to attach key guidelines to each pathway for reference. For example, in the care of the dying pathway, reference guidelines[11,12] would include the following:

1 converting oral morphine to the subcutaneous route
2 prescribing anti-cholinergic drugs for respiratory tract secretions
3 prescribing medication for terminal agitation.

These guidelines that are agreed upon by the team (which should be approved by the appropriate community drug and therapeutics group with input from the local hospice/palliative care services) are then available to all healthcare professionals involved in the patient's care. This includes new members of staff and locum agencies.

## Variation from the pathway

One of the criticisms voiced against the ICP is that it is a rigid format that does not allow for individualised care. If this were the case, then ICPs would have a limited role in palliative care. In order to address this issue it is important to understand the role of 'variances'. A variance when used in the context of ICPs is a variation from the identified ICP plan of care.

Variance can be either avoidable or unavoidable. For example, in initial assessment of the ICP for the dying patient, goal 5 is to 'ensure that the relative(s) understands that the patient is dying'. If this is not achieved by the healthcare professional, it is recorded as a variance, and the reasons why the outcome was not achieved is also recorded. An unavoidable variance would occur if the patient had no relatives. A potentially avoidable variance could arise if the healthcare professional did not feel confident about discussing death and dying with the relatives.

## Information generated from ICPs and the feedback loop

There are a number of ways in which ICPs can be analysed. It is important for an organisation implementing ICPs to identify adequate resources for analysis and feedback to staff. If this is not achieved, staff completing the ICPs will lose enthusiasm, as they will see no benefit to patient care by completing the ICPs. Analysis includes overall level of achievement of goals followed by either full or selective analysis of variance. For example, in the case of the goal of 'prescribing drugs', an achievement of 95% would indicate a high level of achievement. However, analysis of the variance in the remaining 5% may identify a small change in practice that would lead to further improvement, whereas an achievement of 30% would indicate a low level of achievement, and analysis of variance might reveal that a major change in practice (e.g. improved access to drugs or a change in prescribing habits) needs to be undertaken.

Feedback to the staff involved in completing the ICP reinforces good practice and enables discussion and development of alternative strategies in areas of low achievement. In doing so, it is a continuous quality improvement programme ensuring clinical excellence.

## The opportunity to identify and facilitate educational issues in palliative care

One of the key aims of specialist palliative care teams is to promote the palliative care approach among all healthcare professionals. ICPs can be used as an educational tool both to demonstrate best practice and to link theory with practice. They empower the healthcare professional by giving them access to specialist guidance and knowledge in the form of the ICP document that guides and informs their care.

If generic staff are then enabled to deliver the palliative care approach, this theoretically gives more time to the specialist services to direct their activity towards education rather than direct patient care. Areas of educational need will be identified by analysis of the variances from the ICPs (e.g. communication skills and prescribing), and teaching programmes can be developed accordingly.

## Conclusion

ICPs are one potential solution for shifting the culture of an organisation to an outcome-based model. In palliative care they can provide a format for multi-professional notes and decrease the amount of documentation that is needed by the team. Care pathways can empower generic healthcare workers in the delivery of palliative care, providing appropriate guidelines and guidance with care at the clinical interface. Analysis of ICPs enables the achieved levels of outcomes of care to be measured, and analysis of variance identifies areas of educational and resource need. ICPs should be seen as an opportunity to achieve clinical excellence in palliative care.

## References

1  Glanville J, Haines M, Auston I. Finding information on clinical effectiveness. *BMJ*. 1998; 317: 200–3.
2  Thomson R. Quality to the fore in health policy – at last. *BMJ*. 1998; 317: 95–96.
3  Higginson I. *Quality, Standards, Organisational and Clinical Audit for Hospice and Palliative Care Services*. London: National Council for Hospice and Specialist Palliative Care Services; 1992.

4   Overill S. A practical guide to care pathways. *J Integr Care*. 1998; **2**: 93–98.

5   Campbell H, Hotchkill R, Bradshaw N *et al*. Integrated care pathways. *BMJ*. 1998; **316**: 133.

6   Zander K, McGill R. Critical and anticipated recovery paths: only the beginning. *Nursing Management*. 1994; **25**: 34–40.

7   Kitchiner D, Davidson C, Bundred P. Integrated care pathways: effective tools for continuous evaluation of clinical practice. *J Eval Clin Practice*. 1996; **2**: 65–69.

8   De Luc K, Kitchiner D. *Developing Care Pathways: the handbook*. Oxford: Radcliffe Medical Press; 2000.

9   Ellershaw J, Foster A, Murphy D *et al*. Developing an integrated care pathway for the dying patient. *Eur J Palliative Care*. 1997; **4**: 203–207.

10  Ellershaw J E, Wilkinson S, editors. *Care for the Dying: a pathway to excellence*. Oxford: Oxford University Press; 2003.

11  Twycross R, Wilcock A, Charlesworth S *et al*. *PCF2 – Palliative Care Formulary*, 2nd edition. Oxford: Radcliffe Press: 2002.

12  Working Party on Clinical Guidelines in Palliative Care. *Changing Gear – guidelines for managing the last days of life in adults*. London: National Council for Hospice and Specialist Palliative Care Services; 1997 (revised and reprinted January 2005).

# Complementary chapters

*See also Stepping into Palliative Care 1: relationships and responses*

- Chapter 8: Gold Standards Framework: a programme for community palliative care
- Chapter 11: The value of teamwork
- Chapter 13: Communication: the essence of good practice, management and leadership

*See also Stepping into Palliative Care 2: care and practice*

- Chapter 1: Assessment in palliative care
- Chapter 9: The last few days of life
- Chapter 10: Terminal restlessness
- Chapter 13: Spirituality and palliative care

# Understanding the needs of the palliative care team

*Angela Jones*

*...investing in staff, is investing in care ...*[1]

> **Pre-reading exercise 10.1**
> **Time: 25 minutes**
>
> Consider:
>
> - What are *your* needs in terms of feeling supported?
> - What does *support* mean to you?
> - Where do *you* get workplace support?
> - Are your *needs* met?
> - If not, identify *why* this might be.

## Introduction

Meeting the needs of the patient and family is covered extensively elsewhere. In *Stepping into Palliative Care 1 and 2* the emphasis is on providing the best quality of care to the patient and family. However, if we are to provide the best quality care possible, we must ensure that the people who provide the care are *cared for*. Therefore, here we specifically address the needs of the palliative care team. To do that effectively, there must be good leadership and management. Just as the practitioner looks after the *care* of the patient, the good leader and manager looks after the *care* of the professional.

*... caring for the people who care for the people ...*

## The palliative care team

The focus of care for the terminally ill patient and family is the palliative care team who:

- provide a resource of expertise
- lead the provision of education and training for those working in other related environments and generalist palliative care

- provide a range of treatment and interventions to address the complex needs of the patient and family
- undertake research to inform innovative practice.[2]

These are huge demands to place on professionals, many of whom often work for small charitable organisations. Therefore, it is imperative that effective leadership and management skills are integral to, and interlink with, a good support network to meet the needs of the palliative care team.

# Need

Need is defined as:

- to be in want of
- the fact or an instance of feeling the lack of something
- requirement
- necessity or obligation
- distress.[3]

In palliative care, the *need* of the patient and family are perhaps easier to define, yet they are often similar, especially in relation to supporting those within the palliative care team.

Need is a taxonomy[4] of:

- normative need
- felt need
- expressed need
- comparative need.

Therefore, how can the need of the palliative care team be considered, in terms of what is required by the team and the individual within the team, to enable the provision of quality, effective healthcare from which the patient and family will benefit? Adapting and applying the taxonomy to address the specific need and problems faced by the palliative care team, or the individual within the team, can be expanded thus.

## Normative need[4]

Normative need is identified by the professional, organisation or a professional body as the required norms to provide a service:

- access to knowledge, skills and competency framework
- education and training with continuing professional development
- supervision
- professional code of conduct/practice and governing bodies
- self-care and support.

## Felt need[4]

Just as important are the needs to enable the professional to work effectively. These include:

- an identified client group
- targeted population including referral and discharge
- a framework on which to base good practice
- effective and meaningful policies and procedures
- minimalist paperwork and clearance of repetitive paperwork
- minimalist meetings and clearance of repetitive meetings
- information and clarity about the role and expectations of the service provider
- information and clarity about the role and expectations of the service provided to the service user
- a clear and transparent system for monitoring and developing good practice.

## Expressed need[4]

Expressed need is a balanced caseload and role, in a climate of increasing demands on the service and expectations on the role of the provider, including:

- the ability to lead the team
- the ability to manage the team
- the ability to manage self and to regularly review caseload
- to have a leadership and management system that enables the identification of stress factors and overload and the ability to approach and have action taken to reduce such stressors being non-judgemental or non-punitive
- clear and transparent organisation, mission, service aims and target evidence and source delivery of service
- an effective and adequately resourced service
- an application of standards of good quality care and care pathways
- a clear and transparent framework to highlight the roles and accountabilities of the professional and the organisation.

## Comparative need[4]

This is the need to compare what one team provides against others in line with national guidelines, and to develop and/or adopt best practice approaches having identified and put in place adequate resources to meet the identified need of the individual, team and service. This incorporates:

- access to national guidelines
- clinical audit to determine outcomes and best practice
- implementation of recommendations and guidelines in relation to clinical governance
- quality circles/significant event analysis
- process of feedback experiences into the development of good practice.

To effectively manage *and* lead requires constant appraisal and implementation of all four points, and involves:

- coordination
- education and training
- supervision
- mentorship
- mutual support.

**Key to all the above is the provision of** *clear, transparent and effective* **leadership** *and* **management, without which the team becomes:**

- demotivated
- disorganised
- undervalued
- dis-stressed.

That, in turn, directly impacts on the quality standard of care provision to the patient and family – no matter how much the professional attempts to a maintain high quality standard of care.

---

**Self-assessment exercise 10.1**
**Time: 25 minutes**

Within your current role:

- List *your* needs.
- Try to *categorise* these.
- What needs to be done by *your leader* to meet your needs?
- What needs to be done by *your manager* to meet these needs?
- What do *you* need to do to meet these needs?

---

## The aim of staff support

> *The ultimate purpose of staff support is to ensure the highest possible standards of care for patients. These standards can only be delivered if there is also a high quality of staff care.*[5]

The care of the dying patient and the family is one of the most stressful situations in which the professional is involved.[6] However, while demanding and emotionally draining, palliative care can be growing and rewarding provided that supportive mechanisms are available and utilised by the leader, manager and the individual.

We need to care and support the individual and team as we would the patient and family. This enables the team and professional to function effectively, and make a greater contribution to the care of the patient and family.[7,8]

The *Charter for Staff Support* suggests:

> *Staff support helps those who care for others to be fully effective in their service ... it involves more than incorporating recognized support systems, or bringing in a service at a time of crisis. Although these things are very important, staff support*

*also involves the creation of a caring and healthy working environment and a culture which is an integral part of every institutional setting.*[9]

Palliative care equates to dealing with intense emotions and being exposed to suffering and death on a daily basis.[10] It is challenging, and can have a detrimental impact on the health and wellbeing of the professional. The dying person evokes feelings similar to those experienced by those losing a loved one.[11] While acknowledgement of these emotions and feelings is essential by the individual (self-awareness), it is pivotal that the leader, manager and team collectively acknowledge this impact if the professional is to remain an effective caregiver and employee.

When asked to rank the relevant aspect of staff support in priority order from a list of 14, the top three provide interesting feedback:[8]

1  effective communication between colleagues, managers and other disciplines (79%)
2  receiving regular positive constructive feedback (63%)
3  receiving regular praise, thanks and appreciation (51%).[8]

Therefore, one should surmise that effective communication, positive feedback and acknowledgement of one's contribution and efforts are pivotal when *caring for* the professional and team.

Types of staff support should include:

- *having a good listener*[12]
- *technical appreciation* – an expert who provides helpful feedback and work appreciation[12]
- *technical challenge*[12] – someone to constructively challenge your approach
- *emotional support*[12] – colleagues, leader or manager who provide unconditional support
- *emotional challenge*[12] – a respected person who asks whether or not you are doing too much
- *shared social reality*[12] – someone who views things similarly to yourself with the same kind of values and priorities.

To determine to what extent staff support is valued and the working environment is supportive and creative, we need to look at the following questions:[7]

- Does formal support exist in your workplace?
- Is formal support available to staff at all levels?
- How do staff perceive the formal support?
- Does a systematic approach to staff development exist in your workplace?
- Are staff involved in improving quality of care?
- How are staff involved in improving quality of care?
- Are staff achievements recognised?
- How are staff achievements recognised?
- Is communication effective between staff, leader and manager?
- What communication is there between staff at different levels?
- Are staff clear as to how their role fits within the aims of the organisation?[7]

## Effective and supportive leadership and management

Good quality, effective leadership and management are integral to quality patient and family care. However, there is a need to clarify *leadership*, which may not always come from the line manager but from a colleague who has been delegated this responsibility.

*Leadership* and *management* are interlinked, as much applies to both, whatever the position in the organisation. We use the term *leadership* to collectively represent the aspects of leadership *and* good management. Good practice and value indicates that leadership is a matter of *how to be*, and not *how to do*.

Good quality teamwork is a primary coping mechanism.[13] Quality and effective care is best administered by a group of individuals who work collaboratively as a team – as a whole. This inevitably involves role overlap and has the potential for conflict in a highly motivated and skilled team. A primary challenge for the team is how to handle conflict constructively and creatively. To achieve this, there must be good, clear and transparent leadership.

Successful interdisciplinary leadership demands attention to the:

- roles within the team[14]
- role expectation[14]
- role legitimacy
- role adequacy
- role support
- role ambiguity[14]
- role overload[14]
- role conflict.[14]

### Decision making

It is impractical to involve the team in every decision relating to them.[15] However, the leader and manager needs to know when and where to involve individuals, a sub-group or the whole team. When the team is not fully involved in the decision-making processes, it is imperative that the decision outcome is effectively and quickly related to them. However, it is *essential* that the team is directly involved when decisions are of a sensitive nature and/or directly impact on their role, function and resources. To be effective, value and support the team, the good leader and manager keeps the team in front of communication – within the loop. Conversely, the team also have a shared and individual responsibility to effectively and openly communicate with the leader, manager and each other.

Deciding who should and who should not be involved in decision making is based on:

- who has the information to make the decision
- who needs to be consulted before making the decision
- who needs to be informed after the decision has been made.[15]

Therefore some decisions will be made by:

- individual team members
- some individuals within the team
- some team individuals in conjunction with others

- the whole team – e.g. developing services, policy, procedure, role and care pathways.[15]

Poor decisions result when there is a failure to include relevant team members within important information. Inefficiency results from including members who are not implicated in the decision process at that stage.[15] However, any issues that involve the team directly or indirectly should be communicated quickly, clearly, transparently and effectively and never be held over when others within the organisation know of its impact on the team.

*To ask for feedback from one's team, and then not act on the feedback, is destructive and useless, and leaves the team feeling undervalued.*

## Leadership is flexible

A team without a captain lacks focus, direction and vision.[15] Within the palliative care team, leadership can be flexible and fluid, based on expertise, experience, and dependent on the problem or task.[15] It must be acknowledged that sometimes other team members have more experience and knowledge. This is important in service development. A good leader identifies key people within the team who have relevant knowledge and experience and takes positive steps to include them in the decision-making process.

The leadership role changes between individuals within the team but the intent, to motivate the team to the highest possible quality standard, and to take responsibility for planning and problem solving, remains the same.[15] To be effective this means avoiding the urge to dictate, and adapt one's style to meet the prevailing circumstance, while maintaining a balance between the pressures of organisational demand, the need to complete a task, and the need to nurture and motivate the individual and team.

## Communication

Effective communication involves the integral ability to:

- *listen* – to what is said/what is not said
- *hear* – to hear what is said/what is not said
- *explore* – expressed or intimated matters that are actual, or perceived as, impinging on the team
- *example* – actively demonstrate the ability to listen and apply the above in practice
- *take quick and effective action* – to be aware of poor communication and demonstrate the ability to listen, hear and implement factors that improve relationships within the team and effectively communicate.

Team members have a valuable contribution within an organisation. They hold the key to information that is valuable to other team members. The challenge is to ensure that information is shared and exchanged in a clear, transparent, efficient and concise way. To do this the team, leader and manager must acknowledge that *communication* is the cornerstone, bringing the pieces of information together to form a whole.

When problem solving, individuals need information about the issues in order to make an informed decision and formulate action. Staff meetings have a useful function in the sharing of information and decision making. Trust in the leader is imperative: even small issues that actually, or are perceived to, impact on the individual's working practice, if withheld to the *next meeting*, can be interpreted as withholding information. This practice can only lead to mistrust, impacting on respect, value and trust.

## Recognising the problem and offering effective intervention

Good leaders and managers assess and evaluate team (*or individuals within the team*) problems. Having identified the problem(s), s/he should then actively seek to bring a resolution quickly and effectively in a caring and compassionate manner.

The following concepts can be *witnesses in practice*. *You* can help *your* team to identify them, and offer effective intervention.

- *Disenfranchised grief*[16] – unrecognised or unvalidated grief.[10]
- *Compassion fatigue*[17] – the suffering of the helper mirrors the pain of the helped. It can result in physical and emotional exhaustion with adverse effects on the caregiver's own health.[10]
- *Wounded healer*[18] – the belief that one's own woundedness and experience of suffering can be a source of healing and compassion for others and oneself.[10]
- *Intimate stranger*[19] – the professional becomes a surrogate relative or friend. It is possible for the caregiver's personal relationships to suffer as more time is invested in work.[10]
- *Caregiver grief*[20] – referred to as the *private shadow*. The grief of the caregiver exposed to multiple deaths and whose grief has gone unnoticed.[10]
- *Soul pain*[21] – the experience of an individual who has become disconnected and alienated from the deepest and most fundamental aspects of themselves. The relevance for staff is for those who may become alienated from their deepest selves and assume a more mechanical, superficial role in their work.[10]

The above should not be perceived as weaknesses but as something that can impact on any individual who cares about his or her actions and omissions in this stressful environment known as palliative care. Issues need to be identified, and support given, to the individual aiding resolve in a meaningful way, while remaining an effective and valued employee.

# Importance of self-care

Instigating a safe environment, where the professional feels enabled to effectively look after his or her needs, is imperative – that is, to facilitate, and actively encourage, *self-care*. The intrinsic components, skills and caring offered to the patient and family equally apply to the individual working in the palliative care team.

Self-care is an important aspect of support and embraces the:

- work–life balance
- engaging and disengaging with work rituals
- use of an array of coping strategies.

Six domains of the supportive role of the palliative care nurse can be adopted to ensure support for the individual and palliative care team.[22]

1 *Valuing* – having respect for the inherent worth of others irrespective of particular characteristics. Look for the good in others and believe in them as human beings.
2 *Connecting* – getting in touch with the individual.
3 *Empowering* – facilitating the individual to do for his or her self whatever has to be done to meet his or her own and others' needs.
4 *Doing for* – focusing on the physical care of the individual – taking charge and team playing.
5 *Finding meaning* – helping individuals to find meaning in their situation – this is strength giving.
6 *Preserving own integrity* – the ability to maintain feelings of self-worth and self-esteem and maintaining energy levels. Being a reflective practitioner through looking inward, valuing personal worth, acknowledging and questioning personal behaviour, reaction and needs.[22]

To be effective, self-care involves the maintenance[10] of:

- supervision
- therapy
- identification of own values
- development of self-support programme
- work–life balance
- stress management
- grief and meaning
- education.[10]

## Supervision

The support, promotion and encouragement of clinical supervision is integral to good practice. It provides a safe environment, with protected time, and opportunity to share experiences, anxieties and coping strengths, and work through emotional conflicts thus accessing support.[23]

Reflection of events and emotions facilitates making sense of them, which informs and encourages learning opportunities. Models of clinical supervision include:

- one-to-one supervision/supervisee
- one-to-one peer
- peer group
- critical/significant event audit
- peer review
- intra- and interdisciplinary review
- closure conference
- intra- and interdisciplinary team meetings.

Clinical supervision forms part of the support network and contributes to the reduction of burnout. Differing models allow for the work demands of the individual within the team to be shared and appreciated by the whole team and provides mutual support.

## Conclusion

*It is possible for senior nurses to function effectively on previous experience and common sense. However, they can achieve and maintain a higher level of professionalism when using counselling and leadership theory to underpin practice. The leadership qualities required to improve practice should be underpinned by the qualities of a good communicator.*[24]

Just as we apply the above to good quality standard of care for the patient and family, similar skills and expertise are needed when *caring for the people who care for the people*.

Good leaders and managers recognise and facilitate good support and resource practice. Understanding the needs of the individual and team is an *appreciation* of:

- the common understanding and direction
- each other's goal
- each other's responsibilities
- each other's role within the team
- each other's role within the organisation.

The need for good, clear, transparent and effective

- communication
- conflict management
- change management
- decision making
- mutual support
- leadership
- management

is *integral to* and *contributes to* the successful team, and cannot be overemphasised. Even with tough financial constraints, good and effective leadership and management, with proactive approaches to communication and staff ownership, overcome many of the obstacles and/or organisational demands.

Each individual within the organisation, regardless of role or position, must feel valued, supported and appreciated. There is no financial implication to this practice: it is the most cost-effective approach within any organisation. The only cost is that of good manners and respect for one another. This can only come from, be reinforced from, and be directed from the top – that is, lead and manage by good, open and transparent example. *Value those who work for you – and they will value you.*

---

**Self-assessment exercise 10.2**
**Time: 15 minutes**

Consider each of the following statements. How do they fit your experience of your workplace? Answer 'yes' or 'no' to each as honestly as you can; a maybe is a 'no'. It is probably best to put down the first answer that comes to you. These are simple indictors of your work experience; there is no need to get too analytical about them.

*The organisation as a whole — your employer, such as all NHS trusts or independent hospitals or hospices*

| Y | N | |
|---|---|---|
| ☐ | ☐ | I know what is expected of me |
| ☐ | ☐ | I have sufficient resources to do the job |
| ☐ | ☐ | I have the opportunity to do what I do best |
| ☐ | ☐ | I have received praise from my boss in the past 7 days |
| ☐ | ☐ | I am aware of what is going on in the organisation |
| ☐ | ☐ | I can participate in decisions that affect my work |
| ☐ | ☐ | My boss has talked with me about my progress within the past 6 months |
| ☐ | ☐ | I would recognise all the executives of the organisation (e.g. the chief executive) if I saw them |
| ☐ | ☐ | What I have to say counts |
| ☐ | ☐ | I have the support and opportunity to keep learning |
| ☐ | ☐ | The mission and purpose of our organisation is clear to me |
| ☐ | ☐ | I feel the organisation cares about me |

### Scoring

The above explores whether some of the conditions for burnout are present in your life. Count your responses to each question and total the 'yes' responses. The higher your 'yes' response, the less is the likelihood of burnout occurring. If you score 100%, you are probably kidding yourself, or you are in denial. Most people who are okay in their lives and work will get around 75%. The lower your score, the more a problem is indicated. In general, a score of 50% or less should be a warning sign of a real problem that will provide a seedbed for burnout. The risks would be incrementally greater if the score were below 50%.

Conversely, each question has an implicit solution. It is important not to get into trying to get a high score on all of them at once if there is a problem. Putting that degree of energy in to it will probably make things worse. Be gentle on yourself. If there are problem areas, set one or two realistic goals rather than trying to sort the whole lot out.

*Remember, it is the overall picture, rather than individual responses, that counts. The intention of the whole is to raise awareness of the situation so that things can change if necessary.*

Reproduced with the kind permission of Rev. Prof. Stephen Wright and *Nursing Standard*. Rev. Prof. Stephen Wright. 'Burnout – a spiritual crisis' essential guide booklet. *Nursing Standard*. 2005. 27 July. **19**(46).

# References

1 NHS Modernisation Agency. *Retaining and Developing Staff.* 2005; www.wise.nhs.uk/cmsWISE/Workforce+Themes/Retaining_and_Developing_Staff/intro.htm

2 Woof R, Carter YH, Faull C. Palliative care: the team, the service and the need for care. In: Faull C, Carter YH, Daniels L, editors. *Handbook of Palliative Care.* Oxford: Blackwell Science; 1998, Chapter 2.

3 McLeod W, editor. *The New Collins Dictionary and Thesaurus.* Glasgow: HarperCollins Publishers; 1991.

4 Bradshaw J. A taxonomy of social need. In: Mclachlan G, editor. *Problems and Progress in Medical Care: essays on current research,* 7th series. Oxford: Nuffield Provincial Hospital Trust; 1972.

5 Stoter D. *Staff Support in Health Care.* Oxford: Blackwell Science; 1997.

6 Spall B, Callis S. *Loss, Bereavement and Grief: a guide to effective caring.* Cheltenham: Stanley Thornes; 1997.

7 Farrell M. A process of mutual support: establishing a support network for nurses caring for dying patients. *Professional Nurse.* 1992; **October:** 10–14.

8 Beeston H, Jesson A. Caring for staff: setting quality standards. *Nursing Standard.* 1999; **13**(36): 43–45.

9 National Association of Staff Support (NASS), Royal Colleague of Nursing (RCN). *Charter for Staff Support.* London: Royal College of Nursing; 1992.

10 Renzenbrink I. Relentless self-care. In: Berzott J, Silverman PR, editors. *Living with Dying: a handbook for end-of-life healthcare practitioners.* New York: Columbia University Press; 2004, Part five: Context and leadership, Chapter 44.

11 White K, Wilkes L, Cooper K *et al.* The impact of unrelieved suffering on palliative care nurses. *International Journal of Palliative Nursing.* 2004; **10**(9): 438–443.

12 Pines A, Aronson E. *Career Burnout: causes and cures.* New York: Free Press. New York; 1988. As cited in: Spall B, Callis S. *Loss, Bereavement and Grief: a guide to effective caring.* Cheltenham: Stanley Thornes; 1997.

13 Astudillo W, Mendinueta C. Exhaustion syndrome in palliative care. *Support Care Cancer.* 1996; **4**(6): 408–415.

14 Ajemian I. The interdisciplinary team. In: Doyle D, Hanks G, MacDonald N, editors. *Oxford Textbook of Palliative Medicine.* Oxford: Oxford University Press; 1993, Chapter 2.

15 Corner J. The multidisciplinary team – fact or fiction? *European Journal of Palliative Care.* 2003; **10**(2): 10–12.

16 Doka K, editor. Disenfranchised Grief: recognizing hidden sorrow. New York, NY: Lexington Books; 1989. As cited in: Renzenbrink I. Relentless self-care. In: Berzott J, Silverman PR, editors. *Living with Dying: a handbook for end-of-life healthcare practitioners.* New York: Columbia University Press; 2004, Part five: Context and leadership, Chapter 44.

17 Figley CR, editor. *Compassion Fatigue: secondary traumatic stress disorders from treating the traumatized.* Toronto: Butterworths; 1985. As cited in: Renzenbrink I. Relentless self-care. In: Berzott J, Silverman PR, editors. *Living with Dying: a handbook for end-of-life healthcare practitioners.* New York: Columbia University Press; 2004, Part five: Context and leadership, Chapter 44.

18 Nouwen H. *The Wounded Healer.* New York, NY: Doubleday; 1979. As cited in: Renzenbrink I. Relentless self-care. In: Berzott J, Silverman PR, editors. *Living with Dying: a handbook for end-of-life healthcare practitioners.* New York: Columbia University Press; 2004, Part five: Context and leadership, Chapter 44.

19 Fulton R. *In Quest of the Spiritual Component of Care for the Terminally Ill. Proceedings of a colloquium.* Yale University School of Nursing. 1986. As cited in: Renzenbrink I. Relentless self-care. In: Berzott J, Silverman PR, editors. *Living with Dying: a handbook for end-of-life healthcare practitioners.* New York: Columbia University Press; 2004, Part five: Context and leadership, Chapter 44.

20 Papadatou D. A proposed model on health professionals' grieving process. *Omega.* 2000; **41**(1): 59–77. As cited in: Renzenbrink I. Relentless self-care. In: Berzott J, Silverman PR, editors. *Living with Dying: a handbook for end-of-life healthcare practitioners.* New York: Columbia University Press; 2004, Part five: Context and leadership, Chapter 44.

21  Kearney M. *Mortally Wounded: stories of soul pain, death, and healing.* New York: Scribner; 1996. As cited in: Renzenbrink I. Relentless self-care. In: Berzott J, Silverman PR, editors. *Living with Dying: a handbook for end-of-life healthcare practitioners.* New York: Columbia University Press; 2004, Part five: Context and leadership, Chapter 44.

22  Davies B, Oberle K. Dimensions of the supportive role of the nurse in palliative care. *Oncology Nursing Forum.* 1990; **17**(1): 87–94.

23  Wakefield A. Nurses' response to death and dying: a need or relentless self-care. *International Journal of Palliative Nursing.* 2000; **6**(5): 245–251.

24  Hill L. The use of counselling and leadership skills in cancer care. *Nursing Times.* 2005; **101**(44): 23–24.

## To learn more

- Wright S, Sayre-Adams J. *Sacred Space – right relationship and spirituality in health care.* London: Churchill Livingstone; 2000.

## Complementary chapters

*See also Stepping into Palliative Care 1: relationships and responses*

- Chapter 1: Learning to learn in palliative care
- Chapter 2: What is palliative care?
- Chapter 4: The experience of illness
- Chapter 7: The therapeutic relationship
- Chapter 11: The value of teamwork
- Chapter 12: Stress issues in palliative care
- Chapter 13: Communication: the essence of good practice, management and leadership

*See also Stepping into Palliative Care 2: care and practice*

- Chapter 12: Hearing the pain of the carer
- Chapter 13: Spirituality and palliative care

# The value of teamwork

*John Fletcher-Cullum*

---

**Pre-reading exercise 11.1**
**Time: 15 minutes**

Consider:

- how teamwork has affected your practice
- how the team was developed.

---

## Introduction

Teamworking has been an integral part of the philosophy of palliative care since its inception, enshrined in its standards and embedded in its practice.[1] The World Health Organization[2] defines teamwork as:

> *co-ordinated action carried out by two or more individuals jointly, concurrently or subsequently.*

It implies:

- commonly agreed goals
- clear awareness of and respect for others' roles and functions.

Individually, teamwork requires:

- adequate human and material resources
- supportive cooperative relationships
- mutual trust
- effective leadership
- open, honest and sensitive communication
- provision for evaluation.

Using this definition,[2] teamwork can be classified as a more:

- responsive service to patients
- cost-effective service
- satisfying role and career path for professionals.[3]

Two predominant stressful situations for professionals are:

- caring for dying people
- supporting bereaved families.

Although this can be challenging, and emotionally demanding, it is also rewarding; providing the professional is supported. This enables the individual to function effectively and make a greater contribution to teamwork within the organisation. However, team conflict and communication problems are often more stressful than working with the dying.[4]

Building team relationships is difficult and time consuming. However, it is time well spent. Team philosophy, building and support are the primary coping mechanism of palliative care professionals but team conflict is less stressful than in other specialties.[5] Teamwork requires:

- respect for each other's expertise and value
- recognition of the reality of role overlap
- ability to communicate with each other
- ability to deal effectively with conflict, anger and rivalry
- sharing joy and sorrow.[6]

## Teamwork

Nurses are used to working in teams. These teams have generally meant dividing the workforce into small groups, each group looking after the care of a predetermined number of patients. This should have led to better continuity of care with one small group of staff caring for one small group of patients. However, in practice this is rarely the case with staff members being moved from one team to another to ensure adequate staff numbers. This approach divides the stretched workforce.

In palliative care, teams have developed differently. This may be due to the way services have grown in the community. Most palliative care services are provided by local hospices and are of charitable status. The team consists of the following; however, the list is not exhaustive:

- clinical nurse specialists (CNS)
- hospital and hospice consultant
- general practitioner
- district nursing team
- health visitor
- school nurse
- social services
- physiotherapists
- occupational therapists, etc.

Teamwork is a central element of the philosophy of palliative care, where team leadership can be a challenge. However, in palliative care, the patient makes the ultimate decision.

Case scenario 11.1 illustrates the breadth of the team.

---

### Case scenario 11.1

Gemma (30), a young mother of three, lived in a small rural village and the children attended the local school. Gemma would take the bus into the local market town once a week to shop and visit friends. Gemma had a difficult relationship with her parents; however, she had close contact with her siblings. Gemma was estranged from her husband who had little to do with the children.

A breast lump was discovered and ignored for too long. Eventually, this was diagnosed as malignant with widespread metastases.

The CNS was invited to contact Gemma by the chemotherapy nurse to help manage her intractable nausea and vomiting. The first visit highlighted the problems Gemma was having living in a remote village with no family or friends for support. Gemma expressed her wish to move but explained her financial difficulties. The CNS started to build the team who would care for Gemma. The general practitioner (GP) was asked to write to the local council requesting that Gemma be rehoused. The social service department were contacted to offer financial advice and ensure Gemma was receiving all the benefits she was entitled to. The children were having some difficulties understanding why their mother was always ill and often unable to attend to their needs. The hospice family worker was asked to visit the children and liaise with the health visitor and the school nurse. The eldest child was showing signs of stress at school and was becoming disruptive; the family worker worked with the teaching staff and offered them support. The hospital Macmillan team was enlisted to give support when Gemma was admitted to hospital. Marie Curie gave respite when things became too difficult to manage at home. The district nursing team played a key role in supporting Gemma, and visited daily to change the drugs in her syringe driver. The CNS visited twice a week to coordinate the team, and meet Gemma's complex needs. Contact with Gemma's parents and sisters was maintained to keep all parties informed.

Here, the growing team of professionals was coordinated by the CNS (*see* Figure 11.1 opposite). However, the lead changed a number of times as Gemma's care dictated.

**Self-assessment exercise 11.1**
**Time: 15 minutes**

Consider the importance of communication within the context of teamwork.

## Benefits of teamwork

The most important aspect of the care was communication between the carers. Communication was pivotal and a core element of the therapeutic relationship, not only to benefit the patient and family but also the immediate and wider teams. Communication needed to be effective, clear, defined and of the highest quality. All members of the team met on a frequent basis with sub-teams meeting more frequently. Collaborative working promoted Gemma's quality of life, ensuring that all aspects of care were addressed in the way she desired.

Convening a meeting of all the carers involved in the care of a patient is not easy but it is achievable. It is possible for one key worker to coordinate discussion among

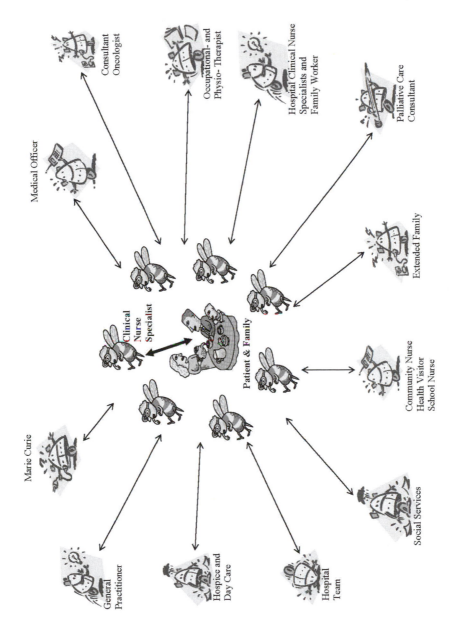

Figure 11.1  The essence of teamwork.

the main carers. A formal framework ensures that attention is given to the team involved in caring for dying patients and their family. In addition, improving and maintaining good team communication facilitates reflective practice.

---

**Self-assessment exercise 11.2**
**Time: 15 minutes**

1 Think about how the team functions when communication is:

- good, clear and effective
- poor, unclear and ineffective.

2 How do these provide benefits or challenges for the:

- team
- patient
- family?

---

## Open communication

The needs of the whole person should be met. The philosophy is from a religious and nursing base rather than medicine.[7]

Teamwork facilitates collaborative patient-led care to the highest quality standards, thus enhancing continuity. By making decisions about care in discussion, the team are committed to improving care and its delivery. However, the patient is not the only beneficiary of teamwork. If the team communicates openly and honestly, collectively and individually, all gain confidence and knowledge to enhance future practice.

## Open relationships

Open relationships provide support for each other, and allow differences of opinion to be dealt with, without problems becoming personalised. The opportunity for genuine consultation and collaboration offers great benefit for the patient. However, the concept of who has the final say, when conflict arises, presents difficulties. In such circumstances, the patient is the *final decision-maker* (the expert patient) who uses many pieces of information, sources of support and their own values as a guide.[5]

# Management in practice

To achieve effective teamwork, managers and leaders must be prepared to relinquish control and encourage self-directed decision making and problem solving. The managers *influence* the situation rather than control it.[8] By managing staff, while allowing them to manage patient care, the team grows in the knowledge that their judgement is trusted. This trust becomes mutual and helps the team appreciate managerial restraints, e.g. financial limits, which are imposed on the organisation.

# Multidisciplinary teamwork

The features of multidisciplinary teams are clear in clinical practice but leadership is often hierarchical.[7] Clinicians work as 'wedges in a pie', each with a defined place in the overall care of the patient, contributing their expertise.

The benefit of multidisciplinary teamwork is demonstrated where a patient is referred to the palliative care team for management of a specific symptom but benefits enormously from the holistic approach (*see* Case scenario 11.2).[9]

---

**Case scenario 11.2**

Richard (42), referred for relief of back pain, found his pain being managed by the palliative care team while the mental health team, who also supported his family, treated his depression. He had the input of a nutritionist who helped him adjust to a gastrostomy and a social worker who both assisted with equipment in the home and gave him advice about an advance directive, truly looking after the physical and spiritual person. However, the reality of multi-disciplinary teamwork is questioned, as the most important member of the team must be the patient, who is often ignored and excluded from decision making.[10] In practice, the patient is rarely, if ever, in attendance at the team meetings. Their views are introduced by a professional acting as advocate. Self-management in palliative care is essential and an important new direction for the speciality.

---

# Interdisciplinary teamwork

As palliative care evolves, there must be interdisciplinary teamwork, where team members work interdependently, and share information, with task-dependent leadership, based on the patient's situation.[7]

Interdisciplinary function is the aim of specialist palliative care teams. The team shares information and works interdependently. Leadership is task-dependent,[11] with tasks defined by the individual patient's situation. The analogy of the hand is appropriate: individual digits of differing ability, function and dexterity work together to achieve more than the sum of the individual fingers.[12]

The synergy created by these teams is beneficial to the patient, family and team. It requires the interaction of the team to produce the final product.[7] For a team to function in an effective way, the members must have:

- a common purpose
- an understanding of the role of the other
- the ability to pool resources.[13]

*The dynamics of the workplace play a major role in a practitioner's sense of wellbeing.*[7]

## Team evolution

When developing the interdisciplinary team, it is important to identify different strengths in the individual members. Moreover, it is essential to respect the individual weaknesses and work to improve these.[7] Interdisciplinary teams produce new challenges, each discipline needing to respect the skills of others, recognising the inevitable overlap of skills. There has to be an acknowledgement of skills that are common to each, e.g.:

- A social worker may have a higher level of understanding of counselling skills but, in some circumstances, the nurses' skills are sufficient.
- A nurse may have skills in teaching breathing exercises but will require the help of a physiotherapist for complex symptoms.

The recognition of these skills, and the acceptance of individual limitations, further reinforce the feelings of trust among the team.

It is accepted that a team requires a range of different roles and personalities to make it work effectively. There are nine different roles, all with positive qualities and allowable weaknesses.[14]

- coordinator
- shaper
- plant
- monitor evaluator
- resource investigator
- team worker
- implementer
- completer finisher
- specialist.

## Team trust

There is an identified need to seek and receive support and accept one's own feelings. Being able to trust another, and talk openly of one's feelings and experience, is essential.[15] Building trust is crucial to the team, and can only be achieved when there is a sense of security for each team member.

Each individual has the right to be treated with respect as intelligent, capable and equal human beings, e.g.:

- healthcare assistants should be acknowledged for the skills, knowledge and experience in areas such as manual handling
- medical officers should be able to question, in a safe environment, without feeling that they should have all the answers.

Organisational attitude is crucial to the success of the team. The team need to be aware of the organisation's acceptance of the effect of stress. Each individual should be encouraged to express his or her concerns without fear of stigma or reprisal.

It is important to demonstrate that teamwork is valued. This means that each individual has to feel valued. The team can be compared to a football team – illustrating the need for different roles to work together, each reliant on the other to produce a positive result.[16] In nursing, the charge nurse could be the captain or coach, the staff nurse being the shaper or forward, and so on. The team captain plays in any position and may fill many over a period, leading by example and acting as a role model. S/he must be prepared to pass the ball (hand over leadership) to the best player who can advance the team advantage and achieve the (patient's) chosen goal. This model of teamwork is demonstrated in this comparison of teamwork to a formation of flying geese.[17]

> *As each goose flaps its wings, it creates uplift for the following birds. By flying in a V formation the whole flock adds 71% greater range than if they flew alone. When the lead goose tires he falls back and another takes over. The geese at the back 'honk' to encourage those ahead. When a goose gets sick or wounded two geese drop out and follow it down to help protect it. They stay with it until the goose dies or is able to fly again.[17]*

## Evidence of outcomes

Evidence suggests that the best treatment outcomes are achieved by contact with a team that is least hierarchal, and shows the greatest collegiality.[18] There is less duplication and fragmentation of care when the team works effectively. Patients benefit from greater cooperation, coordination and collaboration.

# Eleven values of good quality teamwork

## Humour

There is a defined link between humour and good health, reduction of stress and creativity. Humour in the workplace:

- improves productivity, customer service and morale
- reduces sickness and stress
- increases creativity
- strengthens teamwork
- enhances communication.

The power of humour:

- teaches
- inspires
- motivates.

Humour is effective as a:

- *'best medicine'* – laughing for the health of it
- *stress buster* – smiling to reduce stress
- *creative spark* – stimulates brain power
- *teaching aid* – use humour to reach your audience more effectively.

However, there is a need to manage inappropriate humour by setting limits to what is not funny.

## Approachability

It is important that colleagues feel one is approachable. The freedom to discuss not only service and team development, but also concerns and problems, and openly ask for help is essential.

## Identifying the needs of others

Individually, team members need to be open minded that others might not have the same expertise or coping skills. Offering help, guidance and support, *before it is requested*, is pivotal to skilled teamwork.

## Confidence and trust

Confidence and trust is a hard-earned, but essential, individual characteristic of the successful team. All participants must be inclusive of this team principle.

## Enjoyment of work

It is 'okay' to enjoy one's work, even in palliative care when dealing with death and dying. There is much satisfaction in making someone more comfortable, or relieving pain. Acknowledging that work is enjoyable, and sharing that with others, is okay.

## Practice sessions

It is advantageous to hold formal practice meetings, at least monthly, where the team, and individuals within the team, can openly reflect on the quality standard of care and practice. The aim is to constructively develop good practice and to learn from experience without destructive criticism.

## Debriefing

While time consuming, the benefits outweigh the few minutes spent ensuring that, at the start and end of each shift, each individual feels all right, and can freely discuss issues of concern, and not carry this home or into the workplace.

## Team building

The annual 'away-days' have a strong place in effective teamwork. The team meets, off-site, unencumbered by the workplace demands and expectations. The aim is to review how the team works together and how this could be improved and developed and to strengthen workplace relationships.

## Gossip and self-discipline

It is destructive and bad practice for the team or individuals to talk about a colleague outwith his or her presence. This should not be encouraged or accepted. Each individual should hold his or her own court.

## Respect

Feeling of team respect is essential. Each individual should feel valued and cared for. Sadly, while great emphasis is correctly placed on the value and care of patients and family, we are often destructive in valuing and caring for our colleagues. Respect is earned by maintaining the values and practices outlined here.

## Time out

No matter how dedicated one is, sometimes we need to take 5 minutes for ourselves during the working day. It permits the gathering of thoughts and emotions and/or puts into perspective something that has impinged upon us during the shift. It clears one's head. Colleagues should expect, respect, accept and reciprocate this individual need. There should be no shame or guilt attached to taking 5 minutes to oneself.

# Conclusion

Creating a team is hard work. Weaknesses can, at times, be difficult to accept and individual strength can sometimes appear overwhelming. Overcoming perceived professional differences and hierarchy is essential. These can be overpowering and destructive. Ensuring problems are discussed openly, without issues becoming personal, requires patience and skill on the part of team and appointed team leader. Leading an effective team does not negate the need for team management, and compromise has to be truly acceptable to individual players. With the will of each individual, teamwork is effective and successful as long as each remembers that it is the patient who truly leads the team.

---

**Self-assessment exercise 11.3**
**Time: 25 minutes**

Reflect on your understanding of good teamwork:

1    What individual qualities make good teamwork?
2    What impact does teamwork have on you?
3    What vision do you have in terms of promoting cohesive teamwork?
4    Consider how teamwork could be improved in your workplace.

---

**Self-assessment exercise 11.4**
**Time: 15 minutes**

Consider each of the following statements. How do they fit your experience of your workplace? Answer 'yes' or 'no' to each as honestly as you can; a maybe is a 'no'. It is probably best to put down the first answer that comes to you. These are simple indicators of your work experience; there is no need to get too analytical about them.

*Your immediate team – the group of people you work with on a regular basis, such as a ward, clinic or community*

Y    N

☐    ☐    Although our work is serious and hard, my team laughs easily and plays hard.

☐    ☐    I feel able to ask my team for help when I need it.

☐    ☐    In my team, people offer help without needing to be asked.

☐    ☐    I trust my team to keep a confidence about me.

☐    ☐    Work is a pleasure with this team.

☐    ☐    We talk about our practice and reflect on it to make care better, in formal sessions, at least monthly.

☐    ☐    We have pre-shift and post-shift debriefings to check that everyone arrives at and leaves work feeling okay.

☐    ☐    We have at least 1 day a year as a team out of the work situation, where as many as possible of us gather to review how we work together and see how we might improve our relationships.

☐    ☐    I feel confident that my team does not gossip about me when my back is turned.

☐    ☐    I do not gossip about my team members in their absence.

☐    ☐    I feel respected in my team.

☐    ☐    I have the opportunity to 'take five' and gather myself without being made to feel guilty or shamed.

### Scoring

The above explores whether some of the conditions for burnout are present in your life. Count your responses to each question and total the 'yes' responses. The higher your 'yes' response, the less is the likelihood of burnout occurring. If you score 100%, you are probably kidding yourself, or you are in denial. Most people who are okay in their lives and work will get around 75%. The lower your score, the more a problem is indicated. In general, a score of 50% or less should be a warning sign of a real problem that will provide a seedbed for burnout. The risks would be incrementally greater if the score were below 50%.

Conversely, each question has an implicit solution. It is important not to get in to trying to get a high score on all of them at once if there is a problem. Putting that degree of energy into it will probably make things worse. Be gentle on yourself. If there are problem areas, set one or two realistic goals rather than trying to sort the whole lot out.

*Remember, it is the overall picture, rather than individual responses, that counts. The intention of the whole is to raise awareness of the situation so that things can change if necessary.*

Reproduced with the kind permission of Rev. Prof. Stephen Wright and *Nursing Standard*. Rev. Prof. Stephen Wright. 'Burnout – a spiritual crisis' essential guide booklet. *Nursing Standard*. 2005. 27 July. 19(46).

# References

1   Palliative Care Australia. *Standards for Palliative Care Provision*, 3rd edition. Canberra: Palliative Care Australia; 1999.
2   Kekki P. *Teamwork in Primary Healthcare*. Geneva: World Health Organization; 1990.
3   British Medical Association. Health Policy and Economic Research Unit. *Teamwork in Primary Care*. London: British Medical Association; July 1999.
4   Vachon MLS. Recent research into staff stress in palliative care. *European Journal of Palliative Care*. 1997: 4(3): 99–103.
5   Vachon MLS. Staff stress in hospice – palliative care: a review. *Palliative Medicine*. 1995: **9**: 91–122.
6   Vachon MLS. What makes a team. *Palliative Care Today*. 1996; **5**(3): 34–35.
7   Crawford GB, Price SD. Team working: palliative care as a model of interdisciplinary practice. *eMJA*. 2003; **179**(6) (Suppl): 532–534.
8   Miller DA, editor. *Leading an Empowered Organisation*. Minneapolis: Creative Healthcare Management; 2002, p. 13.
9   Lapham C, Laraway R. The value of multidisciplinary teamwork in palliative care. *Oncology*. 2003; **May/June**: 46.
10   Corner J. The multidisciplinary team – fact or fiction. *European Journal of Palliative Care*. 2003; **10**(2): 10–13 Suppl.
11   Cummings I. The interdisciplinary team. In: Doyle D, Hanks GW, MacDonald N, editors. *Oxford Textbook of Palliative Medicine*. Oxford: Oxford University Press; 1998.
12   Parker GM. *Cross-functional Teams; working with allies, enemies and other strangers*. San Francisco: Jossey-Bass Publishers; 1994, pp. 7, 31–40.
13   Gilmore M, Bruce N, Hunt M. *The Work of the Nursing Team in General Practice*. London: Council for the Education and Training of Health Visitors; 1974.
14   Belbin H. *Management Teams: why they succeed or fail*. Oxford: Butterworth Heinemann; 1981.
15   Nichols K, Jenkinson J. *Leading a Support Group*. London: Chapman and Hall; 1991.
16   Powell H, Kwiatek E, Murray G. *The Ward Manager's Premier League Nursing Management*. June 2005; **12**(3): 12–15.
17   Anon. Lesson from geese. www.cuttyhunkrose.com.
18   Feigel SM, Schmitt MH. Interdisciplinary health teams: its measurement and its effect. *Social Science on Medicine*. 1979; **31a**: 217–229. As cited in: British Medical Association. *Teamwork in Primary Care*. London: British Medical Association; 1999. www.bma.org.uk/ap.nsf/Content/Teamwork+in+primary+care.

# To learn more

• Adair J. *Effective Team Building*. London: Pan; 1993.
• Hunt J. *Managing People at Work: a manager's guide to behaviour in organisations*, 3rd edition. London: McGraw Hill; 1992.
• Marquis BL, Huston CJ. *Leadership Roles and Management Functions in Nursing*. London: Williams and Wilkins; 2003.

# Complementary chapters

*See also Stepping into Palliative Care 1: relationships and responses*

- Chapter 8: Gold Standards Framework: a programme for community palliative care
- Chapter 10: Understanding the needs of the palliative care team
- Chapter 12: Stress issues in palliative care
- Chapter 13: Communication: the essence of good practice, management and leadership

*See also Stepping into Palliative Care 2: care and practice*

- Chapter 13: Spirituality and palliative care

# Stress issues in palliative care

*Robin Davidson*

---

**Pre-reading exercise 12.1**
**Time: 15 minutes**

A few months ago, a colleague confided in you that she was agitated, sleepless and often tearful in the evenings after work. She is a community-based palliative care nurse and said that in recent weeks three patients, to whom she had been very close, died prematurely. These people were all around the age of her elder sister who died of cancer some 5 years previously. She was drinking too heavily and becoming socially withdrawn and was about to hand in her resignation. How did you deal with the situation?

    See if this chapter influences your approach.

---

## Introduction

Professionals in health and social care are often hesitant to admit to feeling stressed because of a fear of being labelled weak, unable to cope or incapable of professional practice. It is important that the professional can understand and detect stress among themselves and colleagues. While about 90% of patients spend some time in hospital during their last year, only about half of all deaths occur there. Preferred place of death among bereaved carers is generally home rather than hospital. Approximately two-thirds of patients who choose to die at home receive formal, regular care from community nurse teams and other healthcare professionals.[1]

The sources and effects of stress among professional community carers have been investigated extensively over the past decade. However, there has not been a particular theme to this work and for a number of reasons it is at times difficult to draw definitive conclusions, i.e.:

- Most research has not been based on any particular theoretical framework of occupational stress. Studies have compared a health service sample with a matched control group or normative test data.
- There have been very few studies which have employed multivariate methodology in order to elucidate how the various causes and effects of stress interrelate. Little use has been made of qualitative research methods.
- There has been a wide variety of scales used to assess components of stress. Some are profession-specific (e.g. the Nurse Stress Index); others (e.g. the General Health Questionnaire or the Hospital Anxiety and Depression Scale) measure

psychological morbidity. Sometimes personality scales, like the 16PF, have been employed, as have specific instruments, e.g. the Coping with Death Scale.

Generally, studies conclude that healthcare professionals show greater levels of stress than matched groups of other workers. However, the variety of instruments used in this research has meant that there have been some problems with consistency across studies. Additionally, there are some contradictory findings. This chapter aims to outline a theoretical framework of occupational stress to assist our interpretation of the research. This will be followed by an outline of the sources and effects of stress within a palliative care working environment. The final section outlines some methods that have been used to develop support systems within palliative care.

## Stress and burnout

The concept of stress has been employed in a number of ways. Sometimes it has been used to describe the threats and challenges that confront us. Other times it is said to be the response to such challenges. However, most workers would now say that the response of stress arises when the demands of our environment exceed the personal and social resources at an individual's disposal. The stress response is multifactorial, including physiological, cognitive, behavioural and affective components.

- *Physiological* – activity in the sympathetic nervous system increases heart rate and respiration, and diverts blood to the muscles which may be needed for the 'fight or flight' reaction. Constant stress can produce psychosomatic pain, fatigue or insomnia.
- *Cognitive* – sequelae include excessive worry, racing thoughts, low self-confidence or a sense of hopelessness.
- *Behavioural* – e.g. social withdrawal or excessive alcohol, nicotine or drug use can be used to compensate.
- *Affective* – disturbance may eventually lead to clinically significant anxiety or depression.

It is acknowledged that stress plays an aetiological role in the entire spectrum of physical illnesses from the common cold to cancer. A major meta-analysis which reviewed the literature relating to coronary heart disease, asthma, ulcers, arthritis and headaches found stress to be a significant risk factor.[2]

A useful theoretical model is the person/environment fit. This model articulates the interaction between the personal risk factors and the work environment in which the individual finds him or herself. In the model, stress is viewed as a person/situation transaction. Features of the situation and characteristics of the person combine to influence how particular stressors affect the individual. This model is outlined in Figure 12.1.

As the concept of stress is all-encompassing, it is also useful to think in terms of *burnout* for a number of reasons.

- Burnout is limited to sources of stress in the individual's workplace.
- Burnout among health professionals has been particularly well researched.
- Burnout is more precisely defined than stress.

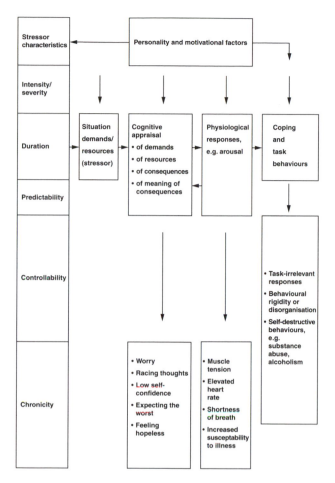

**Figure 12.1**   Person/environment fit model.

The three components and characteristics of burnout are:

- *emotional exhaustion* – wearing out, depletion of emotional resources, loss of energy, debilitation, fatigue
- *depersonalisation* – negative, callous, excessively detached towards other people, loss of idealism, irritability
- *reduced personal accomplishment* – reduction in self-confidence, low productivity, poor morale, inability to cope.[3]

Burnout is a chronic condition that can lead to deterioration in the quality of care the individual provides for the patient. This may be a consequence of lowered morale, absenteeism, poor physical health or an increase in marital or family problems.

# Job risk factors

The importance of the interaction between personal and environmental variables is highlighted in life events literature. It is not the number of life events that predict a stress response, but rather how we perceive the events that determines their stressfulness. Divorce may be traumatic for one person and blessed relief for another. Individual factors like degree of control, personal coping strategies and the extent of social support interact with and can attenuate potential sources of work-related stress. Nonetheless, there are a number of factors which enable us to classify work stressors in healthcare environments. These are relationship, task and system/management dimensions (*see* Box 12.1).

---

**Box 12.1   Job-related stress dimensions**

1 Relationships
   - Communication problems with managers
   - Lack of team work
   - Conflict with colleagues

2 Tasks
   - Difficult patient groups
   - Role ambiguity
   - Role conflict
   - Low sense of autonomy

3 System management
   - Inadequate resources
   - Poor physical environment
   - Old equipment
   - Work overload

---

The general literature on stress among health professionals has produced conflicting findings about the key features of a job that are the major sources of stress. Quantitative questionnaire surveys tend consistently to identify work overload as a major source of stress. However, qualitative research, in which doctors and nurses are asked individually about the most stressful event for them in the previous month, suggests the most prevalent are primarily incidents concerning:

- death and dying
- interpersonal intimacy
- problems with colleagues.[4]

Complaints of work overload and lack of management support may be used to mask primary sources of stress like intimacy, death and suffering.
   There is little doubt that:

- a clearly defined role
- higher job autonomy
- supportive managers
- participative leadership

- cohesive relationships with colleagues
- good working conditions

precipitate:

- greater job satisfaction
- increased performance
- higher personal accomplishment
- less detachment.

Therefore, there are a number of consistent features throughout healthcare work environments that can reduce the possibility of job-related stress or burnout.

Some particular job characteristics can attenuate or enhance stress among palliative care workers. The debate over the past decade centres on the relative importance of these additional task-specific occupational stressors in palliative care. Some argue that the general sources of stress contribute more to job stress than those related to death and dying. Others disagree and argue that there are unique occupational stressors in palliative care that override the more typical ones in other healthcare environments.

Palliative care workers may be particularly vulnerable to stresses related to overinvolvement or sustained intimacy in this highly personalised type of interaction with patients and families.[5] Constantly confronting death leads workers to question how the situation could have been managed better. Clinical nurse specialists providing home care have the added pressure of coping without immediate peer support, requiring a high degree of clinical autonomy. The *'accumulated loss phenomena'* have been the subject of some discussion. They are said to arise from continual conflict between the idealised and actual process of death and dying. Primary palliative care professionals expect to alleviate all suffering, which, when this does not happen, leads to the *ideal* versus *reality* conflict. Furthermore, those who work with the dying can accumulate apprehension about their own potential losses. It has been suggested that the accumulated grief experienced by palliative care professionals can often result in burnout, particularly emotional exhaustion and depersonalisation.[5] The incremental affect of exposure to the psychological and social pain of terminal illness may gradually reduce the professional carer's sense of self-esteem and self-efficacy.

However, some studies demonstrated less burnout and anxiety among palliative nurses than those working in intensive care, oncology and mental health. Furthermore, a review of the palliative care stress literature suggests that *'while stress exists in palliative care, it is by no means a universal phenomenon'*,[5] and concludes that stress among palliative care professionals is largely due to the more usual variables, e.g.:

- role conflict
- poor communication
- isolation from ongoing peer support.

Accordingly, while there may be job-specific stress within palliative care, some research literature suggests this is no greater than that experienced by other healthcare professionals.[6] However, there is a need for more multivariate trials to predict the unique outcome variance of different stressors in the palliative care work environment. Moreover, there is some indication that qualitative, single case studies may accord greater importance to issues related to death and intimacy that are masked in the larger randomised controlled trials (RCTs). However, clearly, there is significant stress within a palliative care work environment that must be managed effectively and appropriately.

## Individual risk factors

There are personal characteristics that can enhance the experience of stress among palliative care workers, e.g. literature suggests there are a number of *demographic* variables that predict stress among this group. It would appear that older, married, experienced workers generally tend to report less stress in a palliative care working environment. However, with regard to experience, there are some contradictory findings, e.g. a few North American studies found that burnout was correlated with an increase in length of employment in a hospice setting, while this is normally reversed in similar United Kingdom samples.

A number of *personality* variables can predispose to work stress. An informative study found that people working with dying patients would report less work stress if they scored higher on:

- inner directiveness
- existentiality
- spontaneity
- self-acceptance
- capacity for intimate contact.[7]

Some *cognitive* characteristics have been shown to protect against stress in palliative care, e.g.:

- high self-esteem
- a sense of personal efficacy
- a higher degree of assertiveness.

From a more psychoanalytic perspective, it has been suggested that people with excessive self-involvement who evaluate self-worth solely on the basis of achievement or material possessions report greater distress in a palliative care setting than individuals whose self-esteem is based around helping others. A number of studies demonstrate that traumatic events outside the work setting – like unresolved grief, a history of sexual abuse, or other ongoing family trauma – have been shown to increase the potential for stress in groups of palliative care nurses. Inadequate preparation and training to enable individuals to deal with the emotional needs of dying patients and their families has also been associated with higher stress levels.[8]

## Managing stress

Caring for the carers has only recently received the attention it merits. The costs in human and economic terms of poorly managed occupational stress are probably incalculable. Workers involved with people who have a terminal illness require sustained commitment, empathic understanding and a high level of intimacy and, if they are not supported, will show signs of burnout or illness. Individuals do have a tendency to use three types of coping strategies.

- *Problem-focused strategies* – attempts to confront and directly deal with the demands of the challenge. This involves active problem solving, planning or other types of more practical activities aimed at overcoming stress.
- *Emotion-focused strategies* – not aimed at dealing directly with the situation, but rather at managing appraisal of the stress response, e.g.
  - acceptance
  - denial
  - trying to positively reinterpret the situation.
- *Social support strategies* – the most common. *See* Box 12.2 for a number of options for social support.[9]

---

**Box 12.2   Staff support options**

- Access to professional mentor for nurses.
- Peer support groups.
- Quality circles that assist in the involvement in decision making and teamwork.
- An individual counselling service for those needing more in-depth support.
- Training initiatives to increase awareness.

---

Support groups can be useful, particularly for primary care professionals who do not have access to informal support in their work. Support groups, however, are ineffective if they just become sessions for airing complaints or if they are not properly facilitated. A number of ground rules for an effective support group include:

- confidentiality
- problems should relate to the work environment
- the group should not be used necessarily for personal therapy
- leaders should be experienced in group work.

More generally there are a number of management interventions which can attenuate individual stress. These clearly include adequate staffing levels, good continued education to improve feelings of self-efficacy, and encouragement to use appropriate anxiety management and exercise strategies. Effective teamwork is essential, and it is important that there is a clearly explicit team philosophy, that time is devoted to team building, and that there are informal and formal mechanisms for team support. Within hospice settings it has been found that teams can grieve more appropriately if procedures like memorial services, death rounds or memory books are introduced. It is also important to ensure that staff who may have lost a number of patients over a short time have access to individual support as necessary.

Clinical supervision promotes balanced and effective care delivery, which results in greater psychological wellbeing among professionals. Therefore, the importance of regular clinical supervision to moderate day-to-day work stressors is essential.[10]

In addition to formal support systems, it is important there is a supportive atmosphere among colleagues. In a survey, over two-thirds of a large group of primary palliative care nurses said that '*talking things over with a colleague was the most useful coping strategy for them*'. The purpose of any form of staff support is to ensure that professionals maintain their sense of self-efficacy and personal effectiveness. Self-efficacy is perhaps most important. When confronted with a stressor, the extent of personal control that we have over the situation plays a major role in buffering its impact.

Within a palliative care setting, it is essential to ensure that structured and informal staff support is the norm in order to facilitate staff grief and provide an environment for staff development.[11] Some people actively seek support while others are more reticent. It is critical that a range of support systems is available that are tailored to the emotional needs of each professional in the work environment.

# Conclusion

The consequences of work-related stress in palliative care are significant for the professional, patient and employer. It is important to identify the sources of stress and to set in place procedures for identification and management of its effects. Burnout is not a synonym for stress. It is a useful, global outcome measure. While organisational issues are important, there are a number of specific risk factors unique to palliative care that can predict burnout. These are summarised in terms of the conflict between the idealised and actual processes of death and dying. Without support, the accumulated grief can incrementally result in the signs of burnout.

Within palliative care, some individuals are at greater risk than others are. Managers must be aware of vulnerable staff. The importance of good communication and ongoing peer support cannot be overemphasised.

Palliative care professionals are an important group of health workers. It is essential that we understand the pressure they face and that they are supported to provide the best possible service to the patient. Provided sufficient supervision, training, time and support is available it can be rewarding for the professional to care for dying patients and support the family.

---

**Self-assessment exercise 12.1**
**Time: 15 minutes**

1 Which of the following are components of 'burnout'?
   a Emotional exhaustion.
   b Reduced appetite.
   c Loss of libido.
   d Depersonalisation.
   e Paranoid ideation.

2 Which job factors in healthcare settings contribute to most distress as identified in qualitative research?
   a Poor management.
   b Intimacy and death.
   c Work overload.

  d Role ambiguity.
  e Interpersonal problems.

3 Affective signs of work stress include:
  a Tremulousness.
  b Early depression.
  c Excessive drinking.
  d Chest pain.
  e Worry.

4 Accumulated loss phenomena include which of the following:
  a Personal conflict.
  b Reduced self-esteem.
  c Social withdrawal.
  d Agitation.
  e Aggression.

5 Demographic variables which predispose to palliative work stress include:
  a Younger age.
  b Lower social class.
  c Poor education.
  d Single.
  e Male.

(*See* answers on page 145.)

---

**Self-assessment exercise 12.2**
**Time: 10 minutes**

Consider each of the following statements. How do they fit your experience of your workplace? Answer 'yes' or 'no' to each as honestly as you can; a maybe is a 'no'. It is probably best to put down the first answer that comes to you. These are simple indictors of your work experience; there is no need to get too analytical about them.

*Taking care of yourself at work*

| Y | N | |
|---|---|---|
| ☐ | ☐ | I get a good night's sleep |
| ☐ | ☐ | I eat a healthy, well-balanced diet |
| ☐ | ☐ | I take plenty of exercise |
| ☐ | ☐ | I can talk through work problems with my partner/a close friend |
| ☐ | ☐ | Work does not interfere with my personal time |
| ☐ | ☐ | Other people's problems at work do not get to me |
| ☐ | ☐ | I practise some form of meditation or relaxation regularly |
| ☐ | ☐ | I can withdraw appropriately if a situation at work gets too stressful |
| ☐ | ☐ | I have day a month when I do exactly as I please |

☐ ☐    I allow myself a good read, or something similar, every day, for at least half an hour, that takes all of my attention and is nothing to do with work

☐ ☐    I make sure I get my proper breaks for meals and refreshments at work

☐ ☐    I know my limits and boundaries and keep to them

**Scoring**

The above explores whether some of the conditions for burnout are present in your life. Count your responses to each question and total the 'yes' responses. The higher your 'yes' response, the less is the likelihood of burnout occurring. If you score 100%, you are probably kidding yourself, or you are in denial. Most people who are okay in their lives and work will get around 75%. The lower your score, the more a problem is indicated. In general, a score of 50% or less should be a warning sign of a real problem that will provide a seedbed for burnout. The risks would be incrementally greater if the score were below 50%.

Conversely, each question has an implicit solution. It is important not to get into trying to get a high score on all of them at once if there is a problem. Putting that degree of energy in to it will probably make things worse. Be gentle on yourself. If there are problem areas, set one or two realistic goals rather than trying to sort the whole lot out.

*Remember, it is the overall picture, rather than individual responses, that counts. The intention of the whole is to raise awareness of the situation so that things can change if necessary.*

Reproduced with the kind permission of Rev. Prof. Stephen Wright and *Nursing Standard*. Rev. Prof. Stephen Wright. 'Burnout – a spiritual crisis' essential guide booklet. *Nursing Standard*. 2005. 27 July. **19**(46).

# References

1  Ramirez A, Addington Hall J, Richards M. Clinical review: ABC of palliative care: the carers. *BMJ*. 1998; **316**: 208–211.
2  Freidman HS, Booth-Kewley S. The 'disease-prone personality': a meta-analytic review of the construct. *American Psychologist*. 1987; **42**: 539–555.
3  Maslach C, Jackson SE, Leiter MP. *The Maslach Burnout Inventory*, 3rd edition. Palo Alto, CA: Consulting Psychologists Press; 1996.
4  Firth-Cozins J. Stress in health professionals. In: Baum A, Newman S, Weinman J *et al.*, editors. *Cambridge Handbook of Psychology, Health and Medicine*. Cambridge: Cambridge University Press; 1996.
5  McKee E. Stress and staff support in hospice: a review of the literature. *International Journal of Palliative Nursing*. 1995; **1**(3).
6  Vachon MLS. Burnout and symptoms of stress in staff working in palliative care. In: Chochinov HM, Breitbart W, editors. *Handbook of Psychiatry in Palliative Medicine*. London: Oxford University Press; 2000, pp. 303–319, 435.
7  Robbins RA. Death anxiety, death competency and self-actualization in hospice volunteers. *Hospice Journal*. 1995; **7**(4): 29–35.
8  Redinburgh EM, Schuerger JM, Weiss LL, *et al.* Health care professionals' grief: a model based on occupational style and coping. *Psycho-oncology*. 2001; **10**: 187–198.
9  Hingley P, Harris P. Lowering of the tension. *Nursing Times*. 1986; **82**(8): 52–53.

10  Jones A. Clinical supervision in promoting a balanced delivery of palliative nursing care. *J of Hospice and Palliative Care Nursing*. 2003; **5**(3): 168–175.
11  Bruneau B, Benjamin M, Ellison G. Palliative care stress in a UK community hospital. Evaluation of a stress reduction programme. *Int J Palliative Nursing*. 2004; **10**(6): 296–305.

## To learn more

- Harris PE. *The Nurse Stress Index. Work and stress*. 1989; **3**: 335–346.
- Hipwell AE. Tyler PA. Wilson C. Sources of stress and dissatisfaction among nurses in four hospital environments. *British Journal of Medical Psychology*. 1989; **62**: 71–79.
- Maguire P. Psychological barriers to the care of the dying. *British Medical Journal*. 1985; **291**: 1711–1713.
- Riordan RJ, Saltzer SK. Burnout prevention among healthcare providers working with the terminally ill: a literature review. *Omega*. 1992; **25**: 17–24.
- Vachon MLS. Staff stress in hospice/palliative care; a review. *Palliative Medicine*. 1995; **9**: 91–122.

## Complementary chapters

*See also Stepping into Palliative Care 1: relationships and responses*

- Chapter 10: Understanding the needs of the palliative care team
- Chapter 11: The value of teamwork
- Chapter 13: Communication: the essence of good practice, management and leadership

### Answers to Self-assessment exercise 12.1

1  a and d.
2  b and e.
3  b.
4  a and b.
5  a and d.

# Communication: the essence of good practice, management and leadership

*David B Cooper*

*... about courtesy and good manners ...*

---

**Pre-reading exercise 13.1**
**Time: 15 minutes**

Consider the following:

1 When was the last time you wished communication within or outwith your team could be improved?
2 What steps do you think you could take to improve the communication?

---

## Introduction

'*Effective ... communication is a master key ... it fits all locks and opens all doors to therapeutic treatment and intervention.*'[1] However, if communication is pivotal, why do we often get it wrong? If effective communication is easy, why do we not practise it all the time? If we are pleased when communication has gone well and angry when it has not, why do we have high expectations of others' effective communication and not pay attention to our own?

As individuals, we should know *what to do* and *how to do it* – there are no excuses. Yet we remain bad at effective communication – unless it impacts on us directly. Then we become experts – we notice how *ineffective* communication damages our day!

Here we provide a foundation for common courtesy and good practice that should be part of our professional and personal lives. We have become too familiar with poor communication and easily oversimplify or underestimate its importance. Consequently we miss the value it holds for individuals, groups and ourselves.

Table 13.1 offers the definition for key words used in this chapter.

**Table 13.1**   Communication definitions

| Word | Definition |
| --- | --- |
| Communicate | To impart (knowledge) or exchange (thoughts) by speech, writing, gesture, etc.[2] |
| | To share information with others by speaking, writing, moving your body, using signals[3] |
| Communication | The imparting or exchange of information, ideas or feelings[2] |
| Effective | Productive of or capable of producing a result[2] |
| Intra- | Within, inside[2] |
| Inter- | Between, mutually, together, reciprocally[2] |

## What is effective communication?

Communication in palliative care can be subdivided into seven parts:

1  patient and family
2  junior team
3  peers
4  intradisciplinary team
5  interdisciplinary team
6  middle management
7  senior management.

All are interdependent and interrelated – none stands alone.

Integral to and at the centre of all the professionals' actions is effective communication with the patient and family. It is they who suffer when communication is ineffective. Therefore, effective communication is like the ripples in a pond, flowing effortlessly between each part.

## What is the communication pond?

Water is made up of millions of individual molecules which collectively give water its fluidity. Individuals within an organisation, or interlinked fields, are like the individual molecules of water. Each is dependent on the other to provide the best possible quality standard of care for the patient and family.

Imagine a stone landing in a pond. The ripples move seamlessly through the water until the pond is smooth, ready for the next stone. In this analogy, *you* are the stone – represented by *ME* in Figure 13.1. The *ME* is placed anywhere in the organisational structure. Wherever *you* are in the chart, *ME* is the centre for effective communication. It is *your* responsibility to ensure *your* communication flows effectively and effortlessly through the organisation.

Therefore, effective communication emanates like the ripples on a pond, flowing effortlessly; each professional having an equal responsibility to effectively communicate with the other: each intra- and interdependent. Only then can communication – and the care of the patient and family – be effective.

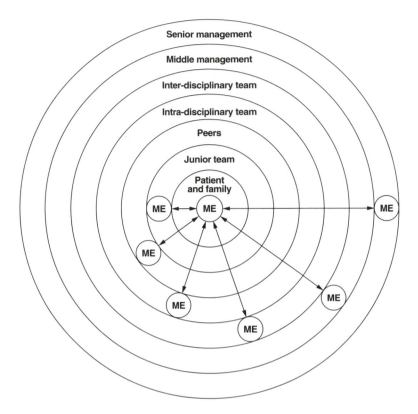

**Figure 13.1** Communication pond.

## Patient and family

The patient and family are central in any care environment. Every action or omission, from the junior member to the most senior manager, impacts on these individuals. Ineffective communication makes the treatment and intervention experience devastating and destructive for the patient *and* family.

The impact of verbal communication between professionals cannot be over-emphasised. How professionals share important and routine information related to the patient and family does have a major impact on the successful outcome of any therapeutic intervention.

With the patient's permission, information relating to past and present health or social problems can be discussed with each professional or agency. Just as important is the information available from family relating to the patient's concerns. The patient may forget or feel unable to express important facts and information relevant to the presenting problem. Often, patients and family can feel intimidated by the knowledgeable professional.

Patients and family can become dependent on the professional. This is not a deliberate act. It is easy to feel *safe* in the hands of a competent professional. The individual comes to depend on *immediate* access and, consequently, sudden unexpected and unplanned withdrawal is disruptive. The patient and family should be informed at the outset about the level and extent of your involvement in their care. This should be periodically reinforced so the individual is aware of *your end-date*.

Moreover, it is possible for the professional to extend contact with the patient and family beyond that which is therapeutic. We gain subconscious reward from their dependence on us – the professional! Clinical supervision aids identification of overinvolvement and dependence. Patients do progress without our watchful eye if appropriate and effective intervention and treatment is managed effectively. We cannot protect them from all ills or dangers. Being aware of one's limitations, intervention and the extent of the therapeutic value takes experience. Close monitoring of our actions is essential. A good marker is when we come to write the patients' notes and we have little to say about the person's progress – it is time to evaluate one's effectiveness.

## Ineffective communication is damaging and destructive

**Case scenario 13.1**

Friday afternoon. Mary is in considerable pain. She and Sam [husband] have travelled 70 miles by car to a specialist clinic. It is a very hot day: the journey uncomfortable and tiring. Both are anxious about the day, the outcome of treatment, and their future. The consultant advises a change in Mary's medication to manage her pain. This is to commence immediately. Mary questions how she should gain this medication and is advised that the clinical nurse specialist (CNS) will make arrangements with the general practitioner (GP).

On leaving the hospital, Sid telephones the CNS, who is unavailable, so he leaves a message.

The time is now 16:00. The CNS arrives at base and picks up the message. She telephones the consultant to find out about the medication change. However, he has already left. She then calls Mary (who is still travelling home) on her mobile to see if she or Sam know what medication has been prescribed. The consultant did not tell Mary or Sam; he merely said that the CNS would deal with this matter.

The CNS telephones the general practitioner and they discuss the best method of pain management to meet Mary's needs. This conversation is based on the limited information available to them. It is agreed that Mary should not be left in pain over the weekend. The GP prepares the prescription and leaves this for the CNS to collect from the surgery at 17:15.

The CNS telephones Mary to advise her of the arrangement. Mary and Sam are expecting to arrive home at 18:30. The CNS collects the prescription, travels to the pharmacy, then continues her journey to Mary's home and awaits their return.

The CNS eventually leaves for home at 20:00, 3 hours *after* her shift ended.

This case took time to address effectively. It caused Mary and Sam considerable anxiety and distress. Throughout the day they were uncertain – anxious – about a weekend of pain. The pressured consultant had progressed through the day unaware of the impact his poor communication and his inaction have caused. Poor communication impacted on Mary and Sam's wellbeing – it damaged them and their confidence in the consultant.

## So what happened?

- Was the consultant aware of how far Mary had to travel?
- Did he assume that the CNS was attached to the specialist hospital?
- Could he have used the on-site pharmacy?

## The solution

- The consultant could have prescribed the medication and advice on its use in clinic.
- Mary could then have obtained the prescription from the hospital pharmacy.
- A standard letter (multiple copies) detailing the change of medication should have been given to Mary along with a copy to hand to her GP and CNS.
- A standard written communication should follow containing specific details.

## Is this time-consuming?

*No.* All involved are funded by the National Health Service (NHS) or charity. Time wasted is reduced. Cost is reduced. Ill feeling between professionals is reduced. More importantly, Mary and Sam would have received effective therapeutic treatment and intervention at the right time and place.

### Be aware of the family's feelings

If you have made a home visit to be greeted by a husband, wife or child informing you that the patient has died, you will recognise the emotional distress this causes the individual *and* professional. Your greeting and response may be inappropriate. If the death is not anticipated and you have been professionally involved for some time, the patient and professional bond is at a deeper level, and you may find the news both distressing and upsetting.

If the patient dies in hospital or home, and you are the professional involved, it is important to visit the family as soon as is practicable. The visit is essential to provide appropriate support and advice, and to commence closure of the relationship in a therapeutic, caring way. There is no excuse for ineffective communication. It is insensitive to the needs of the patient, family and significant others: it *is* avoidable.

### *Junior team*

Students and junior team members often feel isolated from the communication loop. Matters involving the organisation are heard on the grapevine, often half-factual, sometime totally inaccurate. Effective communication with junior members of the team is just as important as in any other area of the organisation. Unease and job dissatisfaction arise when the individual feels that s/he is unheard.

New employees are often unsure of the system and reluctant to express ideas and concepts for fear of reprimand or being labelled as troublemakers. Old hands do not always have the best or brightest concepts. Communication *among and between* junior team member and senior colleagues should be actively encouraged. Where possible, new ideas and initiatives should be given a fair hearing and encouraged. Yes, it may be that '*it has been tried before and failed*' but maybe the time was not right or indeed the motivation. With supervision, support and encouragement, junior team members bring new ideas to the fore that can improve patient care and communication.

## Why is s/he doing this?

The easiest way to germinate suspicion and misunderstanding is to issue a directive that has no prior or present explanation as to its use. For example, statistics – in any format – are the bane of many practitioners' life. Without careful explanation of the value of new statistics collection (i.e. to ensure that the service is adequately resourced and funded), suspicion can evolve to a negative response. '*Don't they think I am working hard enough?*', '*Why are they watching me?*' An explanation offsets the misconception, maintains productivity and improves working practice. Explanations of complex or role-changing information should be *face to face*. It is *not* acceptable to email or send a memorandum – this is, at the least, bad manners and poor practice.

## *Peers*

### Communication upwards: managers are not clairvoyant – tell them!

A common complaint from team members is that the manager does not understand them. Like the manager, we, as individuals, have a responsibility to communicate. Managers do not come to the post with a vacuum-packed crystal ball; nor are they clairvoyant – even if the issues seem blatantly obvious to you. Nor do they know everything there is to know about the workforce as a managerial tribal birthright. The manager needs clear and concise feedback. It is no use complaining that the manager does not appreciate the needs of your job, or that one is working in excess of one's designated hours, if this is not explained to him or her. Likewise, it is no use complaining about the excessive workload and yet still work the excess hours for fear that this might jeopardise patient care: *as individuals, we have a responsibility to communicate effectively too*! And you support your complaint with statistics!

One cannot place all of the responsibility for ineffective communication on the boss! Each individual is capable of demonstrating how effective communication works. If we remain cognisant of the part each plays in ensuring that we are heard and understood, communication is effective and appreciation of each other's roles develops. In addition, each must exercise the ability to *listen to others* and *analyse each individual need*. Having *listened*, no effective *change* is achieved unless we *act* on the information, and *communicate* it to others.

Peers are an effective means of support, supervision and guidance yet we are often isolated in our professional practice. Stress and burnout cause ill health. We can all experience it. It is not a weakness. If we truly value one another, and wish to be effective in communication, and reap its rewards, we would be better placed to support, rather than knock, our colleagues. After all, it could be *you* next time!

## Intradisciplinary team

### Communicating information

Some individuals within teams withhold information. To possess information not yet available to others is often misinterpreted as *power*. Practice and service provision is only effective if information is shared. There is more *power* and *respect* gained by sharing information and resources with colleagues than from withholding it. After all, if no one knows you are holding that information – perhaps on a new treatment or approach – how can your influence and knowledge be acknowledged. Moreover, how can your colleagues improve patient care?

Regular staff meetings are essential to information sharing. If you are a *hoarder* by nature, this will be your opportunity to demonstrate your skill and knowledge, and at the same time, bring the rest of the team up to date.

## Interdisciplinary team

### The admission process

Whatever your area of work, the admission or acceptance of a planned therapeutic intervention with a patient and/or relative is part of your role. To be effective it is essential that professional communication is coordinated. It is often the minor considerations that have an important impact on ineffective communication if omitted.

In emergency hospital admissions, other hospital and community appointments can be missed. Other professionals and agencies involved may be unaware of the admission. Even planned admissions cause communication issues. Hospital admission provokes anxiety, in even the calmest individual. The patient may forget to cancel an appointment. Therefore, immediately the individual is engaged in assessment it should be ascertained what other services – directly or indirectly – are involved, and what appointments may be anticipated during admission. Planned appointments that may be missed, proposed community visits and/or outpatient appointments need to be noted, and each professional colleague or agency should be informed. Approach the family in case they hold additional information. In addition, direct communication with individuals and agencies, by the professional, is essential.

It is often easier to share information relating to your involvement with a patient using a multi-copy letter. It is good practice (and will be much appreciated by other colleagues) to give the patient a copy of this letter.

### The discharge process

If the care needs of the patient have changed since your therapeutic intervention, it may be appropriate to arrange a joint case conference to share valuable information relating to the present and future care needs.

Patients and family feel vulnerable when intensive services are withdrawn. Even though the patient may require no immediate intervention, there is a sense of safety if it is understood that someone will be available to answer any questions they may have should a problem arise. Withdrawal of professional involvement or discharge should not take place until adequate arrangements for the continuation of essential care is agreed and in place. It is bad practice to withdraw a service or discharge the patient without adequate and effective planning. Crises can and do occur. Community services are not always easily accessible at weekends. Ten minutes of pre-withdrawal or discharge preparation will save one or more hours of crisis follow-up contact. In palliative care, the patient may express a desire to go home to die. This may need immediate and rapid response. It is possible to arrange quickly, yet effectively. Communication to the primary healthcare team is imperative to progress a smooth transition from hospice/hospital to home – even in rapid discharge.

It is beneficial if the patient knows the name of the community or outpatient professional who is involved in their follow-on care. This is far more reassuring than being told that *'the nurse will call sometime next week'*.

## Avoiding unnecessary cost and time wasting

Our lives are hectic: full of twists, turns and manoeuvres. Consequently, it is easy to become encapsulated within what *we* do – the task of daily work. It is easy to forget to inform other professionals and agencies about matters that impinge on that individual's day. If this situation is unmanaged then communication breaks down and ill feeling and rivalry ensues. When one is busy, time is of the essence – it is precious and valued. Visiting the patient at home, only to find that the visit has clashed with an unknown outpatient's appointment, leaves the professional feeling frustrated and angry, as if time has been stolen.

For those arguing that this is additional bureaucracy gone mad, the above guidance, if acted on, and carefully followed, is cheaper than the cost of a missed appointment or confusion arising from poor communication. A wasted community visit, or the loss of money due to a missed benefits agency appointment, far outweighs the cost involved in effective communication between busy professionals and agencies.

## What can I do to improve personal communication?

*Common sense, courtesy and good manners form the basis of effective communication.*

Allow for a great deal of personal effort, patience, practice and disappointment, but do prevail. We all have an individual responsibility to improve communication. Think: what would I like from others? ME is the master key. It is possible for an individual, and team, to effectively improve communication.

## *Middle management*

### Communicating change

The middle manager plays a pivotal role in the communication of change. Change in any organisation is unsettling. Half-truth and rumours need little encouragement for dissemination and cause dissatisfaction. It is easier to have all your colleagues on board the ship than it is to stop the ship, circle, and collect those who have fallen overboard. Change affects all members of the intradisciplinary team; this in turn impacts on the interdisciplinary team and ultimately patient care. To share, and be fully conversant with the change and the process involved, can and does lead to team support. Involvement and a sense of being part of the change process, rather than excluded and unworthy of consideration, are essential for effective communication and ownership of change.

## Senior management

> I had to tell a husband that his wife was about to die ... He collected his children from school and I had to tell them [aged 12 and 14] ... It was heartbreaking ... My manager says our job does not entail breaking bad news ... apparently only doctors do that! ... I wish he could have been with me today ...
> (A CNS palliative care in clinical supervision)

Senior and middle managers need to know the detail of the job each employee undertakes. It is not essential for the manager to be from the same discipline but it is necessary for him or her to be familiar with the exact role of the employee. Only then can respect, mutual understanding and communication be effective. Similarly, the manager needs to share with the employee what his or her own role entails.

One can communicate with a colleague and still encounter misunderstanding. Anyone with a teenage son or daughter will know that even when the benefits of having a clean, tidy room have been explained – for the hundredth time – and a check has been made to ensure understanding of the guidance, numerous reminders administered, and the consequences of lack of action explained, the room remains unclean. Each individual can only try to improve communication – to make communication clear and unambiguous. Human nature dictates that some communications will go unheeded or misinterpreted. However, we are not challenging teenagers – we are adults who would like a good working environment.

### Setting the example

During times of pressure and stress, effective communication is the first thing to suffer, yet it reduces pressure and stress. Effective communication frees time to deal with other matters that are important to patient care. Effective communication comes from the top. Senior managers lead by example: only then will the employee find the tasks that s/he is set easier to work with and control. However, a lack of such leadership is not an excuse for one's actions, inactions or omissions.

Direction on effective communication comes from senior managers. If the directive is clear, emphasising that effective communication is important, then it is likely that the practice will disseminate throughout the workforce. However, there is little benefit issuing directives, if, in personal practice, the manager does not lead by example.

## The personal touch

Emails and memos have made life easier for the busy manager. The increasing lack of pleasantries within the communication and the formal directness and abbreviation means that it is hard to perceive the *literal intention* of the message we receive. Managers should be aware of this change and make written communication accessible. Time to include the pleasantries should be spent when developing the communication. Avoid misinterpretation.

## Breaking bad news – workplace

*Never* communicate bad news in writing. This should always be undertaken personally. If you wish to speak to someone about an issue, this should be undertaken immediately. It is poor and ineffective communication to leave an employee waiting overnight or over a weekend wondering if there is a problem. If the matter involves discipline or reprimand, wait until you are able to see the person. If you have to send a written communication, include information about the anticipated nature of the topic. Likewise, if the meeting is set up verbally, involving routine matters, and is to take place in a few days, give some indication as to the topic. This avoids rumour, speculation and anxiety. After all, a happy workforce is more effective than an unhappy one. Moreover, they are willing to give in excess of their hours to the organisation – so why disrupt it!

We have ascertained that personal face-to-face communication is far more productive and fruitful in terms of the manager–employee relationship. It cannot be overemphasised that if the employee you wish to speak to is in the next room or same building and is immediately available – stand up – walk out the door and *speak to him or her*. This will be better received than an email or memo from someone who is only feet away. *It establishes and earns respect.*

## Communicating with a colleague

It is frustrating to feel that one's professional communications and the important issues you wish to raise within and outwith the team at junior, peer, intra-disciplinary, interdisciplinary, middle and senior management are disregarded, unheard or dismissed. It is essential to remember that effective communication is a two-way process. Often information needs reinforcement and clarification. All parties need to understand what is

- required of them
- said
- not said

to keep interaction effective, and the inevitable knock-on effect on patient and family interventions, running smoothly. Do:

- write
- meet personally
- telephone
- email
- fax
- thank colleagues

- respect colleagues
- acknowledge your limitation
- seek help when needed
- understand the demands on others
- be aware of others' feelings
- assume that you need to clarify your actions
- keep communicating effectively – even if others give up.

This is basic good manners; sadly, it is often forgotten!

## Conclusion

*Some people feel that what we do is easy ... straightforward ... but it isn't easy and straightforward for the patient and family ... we have to help them untangle the web of dis- ease they find themselves facing ...* (A CNS palliative care in clinical supervision)

This chapter reflects on a small number of examples of *poor* and *effective* communication. There is probably an almanac of ineffective communication examples that one could describe: each one of us having our own personal story! It is intended to demonstrate that, with a little work from *you* (ME – Figure 13.1), as an integral individual, effective communication can happen within and outwith *your* organisation: *you* just have to give it brain space and effort. It is not a *thing* to do later but an instrument to use constantly – always at the forefront of everyday activities.

Effective communication is cost-effective and saves time. Misunderstanding, anger, frustration, complaints and worry – *for the patients and family, other professionals and oneself* – can be avoided provided we communicate effectively.

Why keep walking into doors? Life is difficult enough! Each individual within and across an organisation has a responsibility to communicate effectively – not just for oneself but for others whose lives we touch in one way or another and who are unable to care directly or indirectly for themselves. *Effective communication is the master key ... it fits all locks and opens the way to therapeutic treatment and interventions.*[1]

*Having cited all the above, none of this holds any importance if the receiver of communication does not listen. This two-way process is imperative if communication is to be effective.*

No professional wants a patient or the family to suffer as a consequence of his or her inaction – yet we risk this every day through poor communication. It is not *their* responsibility – it is *our* responsibility to make communication effective and meaningful to the best of our ability and understanding. If there were just six words of wisdom in professional practice and effective communication these would be:

*Never assume people know ... they don't!*

---

**Post-reading exercise 13.1**
**Time: 20 minutes**

Reconsider Pre-reading exercise 13.1.

- What changes, identified in question 1, would you now change to improve communication in your answers to question 2?

- Has your list changed?
- If yes, how?

## References

1 Cooper DB. The standard guide to ... communication. *Nursing Standard*. 1994; **8**(29): 42–43.
2 McLeod WT, managing editor. *The Collins Dictionary and Thesaurus in One Volume*. Glasgow: HarperCollins Publishers; 1991. Reprint.
3 Cambridge Dictionary online: http://dictionary.cambridge.org/.

## Complementary chapters

*See also Stepping into Palliative Care 1: relationships and responses*

- Chapter 1: Learning to learn in palliative care
- Chapter 3: The cancer journey
- Chapter 4: The experience of illness
- Chapter 5: The psychological impact of serious illness
- Chapter 7: The therapeutic relationship
- Chapter 10: Understanding the needs of the palliative care team
- Chapter 11: The value of teamwork
- Chapter 12: Stress issues in palliative care

*See also Stepping into Palliative Care 2: care and practice*

- Chapter 9: The last few days of life
- Chapter 10: Terminal restlessness
- Chapter 11: Breaking bad news
- Chapter 12: Hearing the pain of the carer
- Chapter 13: Spirituality and palliative care

# Chapter 14

# Ethical dilemmas

*Mary Ryan*

---

**Pre-reading exercise 14.1**
**Time: 25 minutes**

Think about the last patient you cared for with an incurable advanced illness. Ask yourself:

- What were the ethical aspects of that person's care?
- What do you feel were the ethical challenges?

Once you have read this chapter:

- Think back to this person and his or her care.

Reflect on how your thinking has changed.

---

## Introduction

There is a misconception that ethics belong to a rare and obscure field, that it is the province of intellectuals and moral philosophers rather than everyday care of patient and family.

The contrary is the case. No clinical situation is free from ethical considerations. Our approach to the relief of symptoms, and treatment of any advanced illness, include consideration of the hopes and goals of the patient. We have an inherent sense of *wanting to do what is best* for those in our care. We know that there is a difference between the choices of the patient, family and professionals in planning care.

Ethical practice is a natural part of our daily work, not only with patients at the ends of their lives, but in all clinical situations. However, at times of difficult choices – when the right thing is not completely clear or at times of conflict – having a clear ethical framework that encourages logical, reasoned thinking, rather than an ill-considered rushed or knee-jerk response, is extremely helpful.

There are no finite or absolute answers to ethical dilemmas. As science advances and medical interventions prolong life (often using expensive and complex interventions), the course of illness changes, with more decisions and choices along the way. For many people, cancer is a chronic condition with years of illness and various treatments before a clear palliative phase focuses on the relief of symptoms: maximising quality of life. Recognising that life is ending can be even more difficult for non-cancer terminal illnesses, e.g. heart failure or chronic obstructive airways disease.

As well as the changes produced by technological advance, society itself changes in its view of what is right and fair. The ability to stand back from challenging situations and consider all points of view and options is pivotal.

# Ethical dilemmas in palliative care

This chapter aims to illustrate important ethical principles in relation to common clinical situations.[1] Topics covered include the *cardinal ethical principles.*

## Cardinal ethical principles

What is best – for this patient and in terms of resources? The four cardinal ethical principles that underpin bioethics are:

- beneficence
- non-maleficence
- autonomy
- justice.

These are rather daunting words with fairly simple meanings.

### Beneficence

Beneficence means *'to do good'.* All decisions and choices we make for patients and family start with our commitment to help them. However, we can all think of situations when it is not clear what will do the most good

---

**Self-assessment exercise 14.1**
**Time: 15 minutes**

**Case scenario 14.1**
Sophie was on a gap year in Australia when she was diagnosed with acute leukaemia. For the last 3 years she has had frequent courses of chemotherapy but no sustained remission. Hopes for a bone-marrow transplant have faded. Sophie's consultant feels that the time has come to stop chemotherapy and antibiotics although she herself is desperate for more treatment regardless of its side effects. Which course of action would do Sophie the most 'good'?

*Questions:*

- Will it harm Sophie not to have chemotherapy?
- How can we come to the best decision about her care?

---

### Non-maleficence

Non-maleficence means *'not harming'.* At first glance, it appears self-evident that we do not set out to harm patients. However, there is debate about what constitutes harm. Whose views are paramount? For people in the palliative phase of illness, when the whole focus of care is to make the very best of life, the risks and benefits of any proposed treatment must be weighed carefully.

---

**Self-assessment exercise 14.2**
**Time: 15 minutes**

**Case scenario 14.2**
John has advanced carcinoma of the prostate with widespread bony metastases. He lives alone, having been widowed 4 years. His only son is visiting from Australia: he is due to return in 3 weeks. John tells you that he is finding it harder to walk or to pass urine and that his legs feel funny. You suspect cord compression and want to arrange to admit John to hospital for an urgent MRI (magnetic resonance imaging) scan and radiotherapy. However, John refuses to leave, wanting to spend time with his family while he can.

*Question:*

- How forcefully should you try to persuade John to go in to hospital knowing that he risks becoming paralysed without urgent treatment?

---

## Autonomy

This principle possibly helps us most. However, it does have difficulties. Autonomy is from the Greek to *'self-rule'*. It enshrines the belief that an individual's view of his or her own healthcare is extremely important and must be considered. However, it does not give any person a right to insist on a particular treatment, course of action or demand the patient always chooses his or her care. One's autonomy has definite limitations.[2]

---

**Self-assessment exercise 14.3**
**Time: 15 minutes**

**Case scenario 14.3**
Steve (45) a lorry driver, has motor neurone disease. He lives alone and has been a smoker, and was a heavy drinker. He is currently on a general medical ward while arrangements are being made for him to move to a nursing home. Steve, playing his favourite music loudly and smoking in bed, distresses the other patients. He considers any request to change his behaviour as an infringement of his free choice.

*Questions:*

- How do you think Steve's autonomy is limited?
- What responsibilities do Steve's rights to a certain sort of care bring with them?

---

## Justice

Justice means *'to be fair and just'* in the choices we make on behalf of patients. However, it brings with it challenges of limited resources and the requirement for us to use them wisely.[3] We do not have unlimited finances to offer patients the most expensive treatments that bring little chance of benefit. If we make rationing decisions on the basis of need, it is important to recognise the limitations and risks of this approach.

---

**Self-assessment exercise 14.4**
**Time: 15 minutes**

**Case scenario 14.4**
Tracy (26) thinks she has a breast lump but the GP is unsure. She is the fifth young person this week to present with this. The GP feels there is nothing significant but is under pressure from Tracy to investigate. A friend told Tracy that MRI scanning has a much greater chance of detecting early breast cancer and saving lives. For the average GP, this will add many thousands of pounds to his or her annual finite budget.

*Questions:*

- What could the GP surgery do with such money?
- How do you think we should prioritise how money is spent?

---

## *Specific ethical challenges*

Let us look in more detail at seven ethical challenges that face the professional:

1 *Euthanasia* – 'I wish I was dead.'
2 *Physician-assisted suicide* – 'Please help me to die.'
3 *Resuscitation issues* – 'Don't let me die, whatever happens.'
4 *Withholding and withdrawing treatment* – 'If we start artificial feeding how will we be able to stop it?' Hydration and nutrition – 'They are being starved to death.'
5 *Competency* – 'Don't tell Mum. It will kill her to know she has cancer.'
6 *Advance directives* (the adult who cannot speak for themselves) – 'Of course, Dad must have antibiotics.'
7 *The role of the family* – divided: 'I want active treatment'/'No, I want palliative care'.

### Euthanasia – 'I wish I was dead'

Euthanasia is more accurately defined as 'active, voluntary euthanasia', i.e. taking positive actions to end a person's life at his or her spontaneous request. This is distinct from:

- passive euthanasia, which some people consider to be withdrawal of life-prolonging treatments
- involuntary euthanasia, killing someone without their consent.

Many of us will have been asked to help a person end his or her life. The period of dependency that often precedes death can seem pointless and unbearable to the dying person, because of physical limitations, difficult symptoms and the fear of creating a burden for others.

## How should we respond to such a request?

There are several important responses to make. Never hide behind answers like 'Of course not. It's not legal.' The following framework might be useful:

- *Find out more* – ask: 'Why do you feel that way?' It is important to find what factors make life unbearable.
- *Channel thinking* – many people find solace knowing that the time before death which they find so hard to endure may help the family – those who love them – to prepare for their loss. Here is a chance to say and do things that will give precious memories for the bereaved.
- *Relieve symptoms* – as well as sharing what you cannot do (it is illegal in the United Kingdom to take steps with the deliberate intention of ending another person's life), you can relieve symptoms and distress. Relief can bring hope and encourage development of coping strategies.
- *Show you care* – 'You are you – you are still living and, because I care for you, I want to support you in every way possible until your life comes to an end.'

Palliative care, as a distinct speciality, has taken a strong stand against the legalisation of euthanasia or physician-assisted suicide.[4] Arguments against euthanasia include:

- 'slippery slope'
- religious beliefs
- palliative care makes it unnecessary
- motives behind a request to die
- changing minds
- adequate safeguards
- accurate diagnosis of terminal illness
- correct diagnosis and treatment of depression.

One important legal principle that enables us to give good relief of symptoms at the end of life is 'double effect'. Through this, high doses of opiates or sedatives are legally permitted – if the primary intention is the relief of pain or distress – even if an inevitable or almost inevitable consequence of such treatments is to shorten the life of the patient. Therefore, there is no need to stint in the relief of distressing symptoms in the care of someone who is dying.[5]

### Physician-assisted suicide – 'Please help me to die'

Assisted suicide describes the act of a competent person who wishes to end his or her life actively seeking assistance to do so. Cases of 'mercy killing' by relatives or friends often hit the headlines and the judiciary frequently takes a lenient view of such acts in the context of terminal illness and suffering.[6] However, it is illegal to help another person to take his or her life and those admitting to doing so face prosecution.

Conversely, the assisting individual appears to suffer a higher than average rate of suicide, from which one might deduce that helping someone that you care for to die, even when they ask you to do so, brings with it great and unbearable emotional consequences.

In some countries euthanasia and physician-assisted suicide are legal – the latter occurring when a doctor enables suicide, either by supplying medication or information about dosage or technique.[7] The burden of guilt then, if there is one, rests with the doctor.

The concerns about assisted suicide are the same as those surrounding euthanasia, i.e. ensuring we have sufficient safeguards to protect the patient and that we always act in his or her best interest.

### Resuscitation issues – 'Don't let me die, whatever happens'

Establishing resuscitation status is an example of an important day-to-day ethical reality. It is not an avoidable issue. Professionals need to know how to respond to sudden unexpected collapse and sometimes find themselves with a requirement to give cardiopulmonary resuscitation (CPR) to someone who is dying.

In acute care settings, the assumption must be that those individuals who collapse, unless stated otherwise, will receive CPR.[8] However, in the context of terminal illness, prolonging life at all costs is not an appropriate goal. Clear and transparent decisions need to be made and instructions recorded about those for whom resuscitation would not be:

- what the person would wish for
- deemed to be in the person's best interest.

## But how do we do this and why does it seem so difficult?

The Resuscitation Council (UK)[8] makes clear recommendations about:

- a presumption in favour of resuscitation
- respecting the wishes of an individual and their right to refuse treatment in advance of that treatment being needed
- situations including terminal illness in which resuscitation is usually not indicated.

When possible, we are encouraged to talk to patients and jointly reach a decision that respects their wishes.[9,10] Just as we avoid making judgements about the quality of another person's life, especially in the context of severe disability, we should not assume as self-evident the choices an individual will make about resuscitation (*see* Case scenario 14.5).

---

**Case scenario 14.5**

Joan (83) is fit and independent. She is admitted for a routine operation on her toe. Joan surprises the junior doctor by telling him quite spontaneously that she does not want heroic attempts made to keep her alive at all costs – 'Just keep me comfy if my heart stops.'

The doctor would not have dreamt of raising the issue with her, being sure that she would wish for all active intervention.

---

There would be no challenges in raising the issue of resuscitation with Joan. Many people welcome the chance to plan their care.[11]

Particularly for those who are caring for the patient in his or her final illness, it is important to find opportunities to share that the approach to care has shifted from the prolongation of life to the:

- relief of suffering
- preservation of dignity
- quality of life.[12]

---

**Case scenario 14.6**

Micky (35) has widespread disseminated melanoma with bone, liver and brain secondaries, as well as fungating cutaneous disease in his leg and groin. Micky is terrified of dying and begs the hospice doctor to do all he can to save his life. 'You will get me back if my heart stops, won't you?'

---

This is difficult. The Association of Palliative Medicine has explicitly recognised that there are times when it is right not to talk to a patient about their resuscitation status if to do so would cause great distress.[13] This may also apply to some older patients, not because of age alone, but because of the other illnesses suffered by older patients.[14] In the unlikely event of sudden arrest, Micky cannot gain from CPR. However, nor can he insist that the clinical team undertake CPR if they believe it to be of no value. If a way cannot be found to help Micky accept that he is dying, then it is in his best interests both to record a 'not for resuscitation' order and not to share this with him. This would be a better option for Micky rather than subjecting him to an inevitable failed resuscitation with its associated loss of dignity.

Withholding and withdrawing treatment – 'If we start artificial feeding how will we be able to stop it?' – Hydration and nutrition – 'They are being starved to death'

---

**Case scenario 14.7**

Silvia has had a severe stroke and is no longer able to speak or move. She is not able to communicate except by shaking her head. Much of the time, she is tearful and distressed. Nasogastric feeding commenced soon after her hospital admission 3 weeks ago. The team caring for her is divided about whether to proceed with percutaneous endoscopic gastrostomy (PEG) feeding.

---

Concerns about patients like Silvia are common. They strike at the core of the wish to do what is best for those we care for. Key questions to consider include:

- Is thirst a cause of distress?
- Is hunger a cause of distress?
- What is best for a patient who cannot eat or drink?
- How do I care for a patient who cannot eat or drink?
- Is it right to let someone starve?

---

**Reflective exercise 14.1**
**Time: 15 minutes**

*Brainstorm*
Consider the difference between allowing a patient to starve, and an individual's decision to withdraw from food and fluids.

---

These concerns are extremely hard to address. They highlight the limitations of scientific studies with dying patients, who are often too ill to answer such questions. Studies undertaken have indicated that with good mouth care, dying patients do not have a sense of thirst.[15,16] Moreover, patients who are in the process of dying do not to want to eat or drink.

The ethical dilemma is not that the patient is failing to drink, and will therefore die, but that the patient is dying, and therefore does not wish to drink.[17] It is harder to be confident of freedom from symptoms of hunger or thirst in the context of neurological conditions, e.g. severe CVA (cerebral vascular accident) or sometimes motor neurone disease when the patient may have months or years of life left if they are artificially fed.

The Ethics Committee of the British Medical Association (BMA) produced valuable guidelines, revised in 2001.[18] The key points are shown in Box 14.1.

---

**Box 14.1    BMA guidelines on withholding and withdrawing treatment**

- Prolonging life at all cost is not an appropriate goal.
- Voluntary refusal of treatment by a competent adult must be respected.
- Decisions about whether to start or continue treatments should be based on the net benefit to the patient.
- Artificial nutrition and hydration constitutes medical treatment.
- Where patients cannot express their views, doctors must take account of their previously expressed wishes, the likelihood of improvement and the degree of pain or suffering to be endured.
- Team working is vital.
- All proposals to withdraw or withhold artificial nutrition should be formally reviewed by a senior clinician who is not a part of the team.

---

Despite some criticisms, the BMA guidelines provide a clear framework to consider challenging issues, which has been endorsed by the General Medical Council (GMC).[19]

## Competency – 'Don't tell Mum. It will kill her to know she has cancer'

We are fortunate to work in a healthcare system that recognises the importance of a partnership of expertise between the patient and professional. Much of what you have read so far shows the weight given to the views and choices of the individual.

> *Every human being of adult years has a right to determine what shall be done with his or her body...* (Judge Benjamin Cardozo, 1914)

At present, a patient has the right to refuse a treatment – but cannot insist on it if it is not deemed by the clinical team to be appropriate. Even when a particular treatment has been refused by the patient, a duty of care remains including the offering of personal hygiene, and food or fluid if the patient is able to swallow.

It is important for us to know when a patient is able to make decisions about his or her care. This ability is sometimes referred to as 'capacity' or 'competency'. The High Court in England has set out what individuals need to be able to do to demonstrate capacity (see Box 14.2).

---

**Box 14.2    High Court in England**

Individuals have capacity if they can:

- understand in broad terms and simple language the purpose and nature of the proposed medical treatment
- understand its benefits, risks and alternatives
- understand in broad terms the consequences of not receiving the treatment
- make a free choice
- understand the information long enough to make a decision.

---

Competence is relevant to the decision in question (*see* Case scenario 14.8).

Case scenario 14.8

Mary (48) has Down's syndrome. She has learning difficulties and has spent her life in care. She developed lymphoma, with weight loss, sweats and severe abdominal pain. On discussion with the haematologist, it is clear that Mary would wish to have active treatment at present but realises that she has a very serious illness and might not get better.

## Advance directives (the adult who cannot speak for themselves) – 'Of course, Dad must have antibiotics'

Although health professionals can feel threatened by them, *advance directives* or *'living wills'* are something we should encourage and respect. They provide the individual with a means to refuse medical treatment, in advance, should they become mentally or physically incapable of making their wishes known.[20,21]

An *advance directive* is legally valid under common law if it meets the criteria shown in Box 14.3.

Box 14.3   Validity of an advance directive

- The patient is competent and over 18.
- The patient is fully informed at the time the directive is made.
- The patient is not pressurised to sign the directive.
- The directive covers specific medical conditions.
- The directive has not been withdrawn verbally or in writing since signing.
- The patient is not competent to make a contemporaneous decision.

## The role of the family – divided: 'I want active treatment'/'No, I want palliative care'

When a patient is able to speak for his or her self, we must seek permission before having any conversation with the family about the illness. To ignore this not only breaches confidentiality but also creates tension and distance between the person who is ill and close family. In such circumstances, families are usually acting with the best of motives in protecting someone from bad news or difficult decisions. However, this is only good practice if it is the patient's wish (*see* Case scenario 14.9).

Case scenario 14.9

Jimmy (64) is dying from end-stage heart failure. All life-prolonging treatments have been stopped after discussion with him. He has been comfortable and not distressed for several days when he develops a productive cough and a temperature. His son and daughter-in-law stop the GP, as he arrives on a visit, to insist that Dad [Jimmy] be given antibiotics. The doctor explains his duty to talk to Jimmy before making a decision. With Jimmy's permission, the family

> are present when the question of antibiotics, and the likely consequences of not having them, is discussed. Jimmy was content to know that his life was near its end, and clear that he did not wish for any more active treatment. He died peacefully 3 days later.

Unlike some countries, including the USA, relatives in England have no legal right to demand or refuse treatment on behalf of the patient when the patient is no longer competent to do so. The clinical responsibility rests with the doctor in charge. However, relatives do have a crucial role in helping the clinical team to understand the patient, and give an idea of what s/he would want in terms of end-of-life care (*see* Case scenario 14.10).

---

**Case scenario 14.10**

Hugh (22) sustained a severe head injury in a devastating road traffic accident. His parents feel under pressure in deciding whether to discontinue artificial ventilation and proceed with organ retrieval. The intensive therapy unit (ITU) consultant talked with them to discover more about Hugh, his love of adventure and sport and determination to live life to the full. He had spoken some years ago about his desire for his organs to be used and of not wanting to be kept alive if he became dependent for all care. The doctor can then explain the views of the team that Hugh would not have wanted his life prolonged. The decision was taken to switch off the ventilator, 1 day later, after completion of tests to confirm brainstem death. Hugh died with his family at his side.

---

## Conclusion

Ethics is deeply concerned with the ordinary and practical issues of everyday practice. In considering the rights and wrongs of each clinical situation, it is necessary to look at the theoretical principles, to balance the options and formulate a decision that serves the best interests of the patient. Ethical practice is about making a reasoned and reasonable decision, and being open to differing points of view.

For someone with advanced or terminal illness, dying is not something to be avoided at all costs.

*The ultimate aim is the preservation of dignity and quality standard of care.*

## References

1   Jeffery P, Millard P. An ethical framework for clinical decision-making at the end of life. *R Soc Med*. 1997; **90**: 504–506.
2   Farsides C. Autonomy and its implications for palliative care: a Northern European perspective. *Palliative Med*. 1998; **12**: 147–151.
3   Hope T. Rationing and life-saving treatment. *J Med Ethics*. 2001; **27**: 179–185.

4   National Council for Hospice and Specialist Palliative Care Services. *Voluntary Euthanasia: the council's view.* London: National Council for Hospice and Specialist Palliative Care Services; 1997.

5   Gillon R. When doctors might kill their patients. *BMJ.* 1999; **318**: 1431–1432.

6   Wilkinson P. Daughter walks free over 'mercy killing'. *The Times.* 30 June 1998.

7   Chin A. Legalised physician-assisted suicide in Oregon – the first year's experience. *NEJM.* 1999; **340**: 577–583.

8   British Medical Association. *Decisions Relating to Cardiopulmonary Resuscitation. A joint statement from the British Medical Association, the Resuscitation Council (UK) and the Royal College of Nursing.* London: British Medical Association; 2002.

9   Hill M, MacQuillan G, Forsyth M *et al.* Cardiopulmonary resuscitation: who makes the decision? *BMJ.* 1994; **308**: 1677.

10  Randall F. Recent guidance on resuscitation: patients' choices and doctor's duties. *Palliative Med.* 2001; **15**: 449–450.

11  Attwood S, Anderson K, Mitchell T. Discussing cardiopulmonary resuscitation with patients. *Br J Nursing.* 2001; **10**: 1201–1207.

12  Willard C. Cardiopulmonary resuscitation for palliative care patients: a discussion of ethical issues. *Palliative Med.* 2000; **14**: 308–312.

13  National Council for Hospice and Specialist Palliative Care Services and Association for Palliative Medicine (Great Britain and Ireland). Ethical decision making: CPR for people who are terminally ill. *Eur J Palliative Care.* 1997; **4**: 125.

14  Stewart K, Wagg A, Kinirons M. When can elderly patients be excluded from discussing resuscitation? *J Roy Coll Phys.* 1996; **30**: 133–135.

15  Burge F. Dehydration symptoms of palliative care patients. *J Pain Symptom Manage.* 1993; **8**: 454–464.

16  Ellershaw J, Sutcliffe J, Saunders C. Dehydration and the dying patient. *J Pain Symptom Manage.* 1995; **10**: 192–197.

17  Lennard-Jones JE. Giving or holding fluids and nutrients: ethical and legal aspects. *J R Col. Phys.* 1999; **33**: 39–45.

18  Luttrell S. British Medical Journal Editorial. Withholding and withdrawing life-prolonging medical treatment. *BMJ.* 26 June 1999; **318**(7200): 1709–1710.

19  General Medical Council. *Withholding and Withdrawing Life-sustaining Treatments: good practice in decision making.* London: General Medical Council; 2002.

20  British Medical Association. *Advance Statements About Medical Treatment: a code of practice.* London: British Medical Association; 1995.

21  Gilbert J. The benefits and problems of living wills in cancer patients. *Prog Pall Care.* 1994; **4**: 4–6.

# To learn more

- Hope T. *Medical Ethics: a very short introduction.* Oxford: Oxford University Press; 2004.
- Macdonald E. *Difficult Conversations in Medicine.* Oxford: Oxford University Press; 2004.
- Randall F, Downie RS. *Palliative Care Ethics: a companion for all specialities,* 2nd edition. Oxford: Oxford Medical Publications; 1999.
- Webb P, editor. *Ethical Issues in Palliative Care.* Manchester: Hochland and Hochland; 2004.

## Complementary chapters

*See also Stepping into Palliative Care 1: relationships and responses*

- Chapter 3: The cancer journey
- Chapter 4: The experience of illness
- Chapter 5: The psychological impact of serious illness
- Chapter 6: Hope and coping strategies
- Chapter 11: The value of teamwork

*See also Stepping into Palliative Care 2: care and practice*

- Chapter 1: Assessment in palliative care
- Chapter 3: Symptom management: a framework
- Chapter 9: The last few days of life
- Chapter 11: Breaking bad news
- Chapter 14: Bereavement
- Chapter 16: The special needs of the neurological patient

Chapter 15

# Transcultural and ethnic issues at the end of life

*Jonathan Koffman*

**Pre-reading exercise 15.1**
**Time: 20 minutes**

Think about a patient with advanced cancer you have cared for recently who comes from a black or minority ethnic community. Answer the following questions:

- How did this patient express his or her distress?
- Was this similar or different to other patients you have cared for?
- What were your preconceptions about what would be important for this patient at the end of life?
- What was the reality?
- How did you negotiate common ground with the patient and family?

Read this chapter and decide whether you would approach this patient differently.

## Introduction

Palliative care has been defined by the World Health Organization as:

> an approach that improves the quality of life of patients and their families facing the problem associated with life-threatening illness, through the prevention and relief of suffering by means of early identification and impeccable assessment and treatment of pain and other problems, physical, psychosocial and spiritual.[1]

To achieve its aims, palliative care can be provided in any number of settings including:

- hospitals
- hospices
- residential and nursing homes
- people's own homes.

Over the last several decades the experience of advanced disease, dying and bereavement have all significantly benefited from palliative care. However, in the United Kingdom[2–4] and elsewhere[5] there has been growing concern about how we manage these experiences among black and minority ethnic communities.

The chapter aims to provide the reader with an appreciation of the current controversies with the language of understanding diversity in society. It explores the experiences of advanced disease, and responses to it, among black and minority communities, including:

- the influence of ethnicity and culture on symptoms associated with advanced disease
- access to specialist palliative care services
- communication and information
- the contribution of informal caregivers
- the roles of religion and spirituality.

The chapter draws on current evidence, primarily but not exclusively, from the United Kingdom and the USA.

---

**Self-assessment exercise 15.1**
**Time: 10 minutes**

Race, ethnicity and culture are referred to frequently in the palliative care literature.

- Are they interchangeable?
- Do they mean the same thing?

---

## Understanding diversity and semantic confusion

How we understand the influence of

- diversity in patterns of advanced disease
- illness experiences
- responses to treatment
- the use of specialist palliative care services

is important, given increasing evidence that we are not all equal in death.[2,3,5–8] However, in approaching the issue of diversity we need to be aware of a complex and contentious history in the evolution of ideas and terminology used. Semantic confusion is common when the concepts of race, ethnicity and culture are referred to in palliative care research.[9] They are often:

- used interchangeably
- subject to misuse
- confused with other social metrics – e.g. social class or education[10]
- changed due to prevailing fashions and politics.[11]

In this section I define, and critically appraise, race, ethnicity and culture to assess their ability to describe and explain differences at the end of life.

## Race

Race relies heavily on an expectation of biological differences between people and populations.[12] Historically, race has been used to describe geographically separated populations (e.g. African race), cultural groups (Jews), nationality (English race), and mankind in general (human race). Racialised research in science has a long and inglorious history.[13,14] In the mid-19th century, the *cephalic index* – a method for describing the shape of the skull – became a popular way of describing and dividing races. Under the influence of phrenology, a hierarchy of races was devised with white Europeans at the top and black Africans at the bottom. Intelligence, physique, culture and morality were all placed in an order, the so-called 'Great Chain of Being' philosophy used to justify slavery, imperialism, anti-immigration policy and the social status quo.[15] Biological determinism also became prominent in medicine and medical practitioners frequently contributed to racialised science,[16] with the theory of racial hygiene in Nazi Germany being a horrific and notorious example. However, differences that do exist between peoples and populations are minor and largely reflect superficial physical characteristics, e.g. facial features, hair or skin colour. Therefore, many researchers have now discredited race as being inaccurate and misleading.[17]

## Ethnicity

Less controversial, but equally misunderstood, is the concept of ethnicity.[18,19] It has a number of meanings used to indicate a distinct people or tribe, and also those who are heathen. In the health research context it has been defined as:

> *Shared origins or social backgrounds; shared culture and traditions that are distinctive, maintained between generations, and lead to a sense of identity and group; and a common language or religious tradition.*[20]

### The challenge of operationalising ethnicity

Ethnicity is not easily measured since there are no accurate, repeatable and valid proxies for identity.[20] The ethnic groups identified by the Office for National Statistics in the decennial UK census are usually adopted. Table 15.1 provides the categories used in the 1991 census and those asked in the census in 2001. However, over the years, several methods have been adopted.

- Some researchers have classified subjects' ethnicity by their skin colour.[21] But this method is imprecise, subjective and therefore unreliable. For example, an observer could not accurately distinguish by observation alone between Muslim and Hindu Punjabis, who are in many important respects culturally distinct.[20]
- Names analysis has been used to identify people with origins in the Indian sub-continent in several studies.[22] South Asian names are distinctive and frequently indicate religion.[23] This method of identifying groups of people has been confirmed as sensitive and specific and allows both prospective and retrospective sampling. However, other ethnic groups, for example black Caribbeans, share names with white populations.
- Country of birth, as coded on birth and death registration certificates, has commonly been used as an index of ethnicity. It is objective but crude.[24] For example, India

is culturally diverse with many distinct ethnic groups, comprises a very complex caste system, has in excess of eight major religions, and over 15 official languages.[25] Yet Indians are frequently grouped as one by this method, a classification comparable to being 'European'.

Further difficulties with ethnicity involve self-assignment that poses problems, not least since there is evidence that many people change their assignment over time, as is their prerogative.[26] USA-based research has shown that at least 35% of respondents altered their self-assignment over a year and in the validation study following the 1991 British census 12% of 'black' people altered their ethnic group, as did 22% of 'other' category.[27]

**Table 15.1** Ethnic classifications: 1991 and 2001 compared

| *1991 census* | *2001 census* |
| --- | --- |
| White | White – British<br>White – Irish<br>White – Any other white background (please write in) |
| White – other | Mixed – White/Black Caribbean<br>Mixed – White/Black African<br>Mixed – White/Asian<br>Any other mixed background (please write in) |
| Black – Caribbean | Black or Black British: Caribbean |
| Black – African | Black or Black British: African |
| Black – other | Black or Black British:<br>Any other background (please write in) |
| Indian | Asian or Asian British: Indian |
| Pakistani | Asian or Asian British: Pakistani |
| Bangladeshi | Asian or Asian British: Bangladeshi |
| Asian – other | Asian or Asian British:<br>Any other background (please write in) |
| Chinese | Chinese or other ethnic group<br>Any other (please write in) |
| Any other ethnic group | Other ethnic group<br>Any other (please write in) |

## Exploring ethnicity: controversial yet still attractive

Critics point out that 'ethnic' groupings crudely lump people together with different cultural and health beliefs and behaviours and may sometimes be racist.[28] This too has implications for palliative care. The term Asian in the United Kingdom has been used to include people as varied as the socio-economically deprived, heavy smoking, meat-eating Bangladeshi population in east London, and the socio-economically affluent, vegetarian, non-smoking Punjabi Sikh population of west London. This logic is wrong. Another unintended result of categorising people according to ethnicity is that it can foreclose any question as to why certain population groups experience more ill health than others, leaving researchers and epidemiologists blind to the meaning of more relevant local and individual explanations. But denying the value of exploring ethnic group comparisons may lead some researchers to ignore important health-related issues. Many examples can be cited, e.g. equity of access to healthcare has been shown to be inversely related to minority ethnic status.[29] Uptake of specialist palliative care services, discussed later in this chapter, has also been shown to be lower among black Caribbeans and other ethnic groups.[7]

## Culture

Culture is a complex and problematic social concept where a range of definitions exist. Culture may be viewed as *'a totality of inter-related, but often disjointed and contradictory ideas and activities that characterise life of a social group'*.[30] Therefore, culture can be seen as a *'recipe'* for living in the world.[31] It also provides us with a means of transmitting these *'recipes'* to the next generation, by the use of symbols, language and rituals.

Culture as a social construct is characterised by the behaviours and attitudes of a social group. It influences us individually, and at group level. How it operates is fascinating. Put simply, it can be compared to the layers of an onion,[32] or a series of concentric circles that include:

- *Tertiary level* – visible to the outsider, consisting of things which can be seen, heard, tasted, worn, or otherwise observed fairly easily.
- *Secondary level* – only members of the group know rules about common understandings and behaviours. Although these can be articulated in words when necessary, people take them for granted as normal and universal.
- *Primary level* – represents the deepest level where the rules are known to all, obeyed by all, but seldom, if ever, stated. Its rules are implicit, taken for granted, almost impossible for the average person to state as a system, and generally out of awareness.

### Culture: is it an adequate reflection of who we are?

Our cultural background has an important influence on many aspects of our lives including:

- how we make sense of illness
- symptoms
- the process of dying
- bereavement.

All these are influenced by our:

- beliefs
- behaviours
- perceptions
- emotions
- religion
- rituals
- structure
- diet
- dress
- self-image.

However, it has been argued that the culture which we are born into and learn is far from the only influence that determines our world view.[33] Other important factors (*see* Box 15.1), play some part in isolation, in combination, and in different proportions. At times we may act more 'culturally' than in others when our behaviour will be determined by:

- personality
- economic status
- education
- characteristics of our environment.

Further, generalisations about culture are problematic as they potentially lead to the development of stereotypes, prejudices, misunderstandings and discrimination. Another reason for avoiding generalisations is that cultures are never static and they are in a constant process of adaptation and change. It is for these reasons that culture is notoriously difficult to operationalise and then measure.[34]

---

**Box 15.1   Factors other than culture that influence our world view**

- *Individual factors* – e.g. age, gender, personality, intelligence, experience, and physical and emotional state.
- *Educational factors* – formal and informal, including education into religious, ethnic and professional sub-cultures.
- *Socio-economic factors* – e.g. class, economic status, professional occupation, and informal networks of social support from family, friends and community.
- *Environmental factors* – e.g. population density, housing, roads, public transport and health facilities.

---

## Summary

There are no simple answers about which terminology to use in palliative care that help us explore and understand diversity at the end of life. Researchers, particularly in the USA, continue to assume race is acceptable to categorise groups within society. This remains highly controversial. In the United Kingdom, the drive to categorise by ethnic group continues. The danger of both approaches is that they serve to reify '*race*' and '*ethnicity*' as entities that people are born into and inhabit, and are then brought into the social world. This conceptual '*fixing*' of race and ethnicity and the product of its analysis can also serve to produce and reproduce wider forms of essentialism and stereotyping.[11] Novel approaches that help capture people's identities more effectively than any definition of *race*, *ethnicity*, and *culture* are needed.

# The experience of advanced disease: the influence of ethnicity and culture

An understanding of cultural factors is important. They mediate the:

- ways in which symptoms associated with advanced disease are identified and interpreted
- appropriate modes of expression of pain and other symptoms and associated suffering
- whether an illness and symptoms are stigmatised
- whether the dependency needs that accompany advanced disease are considered an acceptable part of the normal life cycle or marginalised.

The evidence of the influence of cultural and ethnic factors on symptom interpretation is fascinating and frequently raises more questions than it answers. A 1950s study[35] demonstrated differences among old American, Irish and other migrant communities' perceptions of their pain. Levels of symptom-related distress among black Caribbeans are significantly higher compared with native-born white United Kingdom patients with advanced cancer living in south London.[36] However, this was only partly explained by simple variations in treatment levels between the two groups (*see* Figure 15.1). It has been suggested that the language of expressing symptom-related distress may be reinforced by cultural expectations.[36,37] Expressions of suffering have been shown to serve a purpose. It has been observed in some African-American communities that suffering is redemptive, bringing those who experience it closer to God.[5]

In other communities, the actual language used to describe distress and suffering has implications for the delivery of palliative care. The expression 'Dil *me* girda hai', used by Punjabis in Bedford, often translates as the '*sinking heart*' to reflect a range of psychological and somatic conditions.[38] In addition, '*generalised hopelessness*', which characterises depressive disorders in women living in London, would not be regarded as abnormal among Hindu, Muslim and Buddhist women who would regard '*hopelessness*' as an aspect of life which can only be overcome on the path to salvation. Ahmed[39] takes the view that while South Asian patients may be well aware of their psychosomatic symptoms, general practitioners (including Asian GPs) tend only to acknowledge physical symptoms, but do not recognise psychological distress. The ongoing challenge is for professionals to explore and acknowledge culturally determined understandings and expressions associated with advanced disease that do not mirror their own.

# Access to specialist palliative care

According to the Office of National Statistics people from minority ethnic backgrounds now represent about 8% of the population in the United Kingdom. Although there is a lack of data about people from minority ethnic communities, what is available demonstrates that some groups experience significant disadvantage across the board, and others experience it in some areas. Minority ethnic

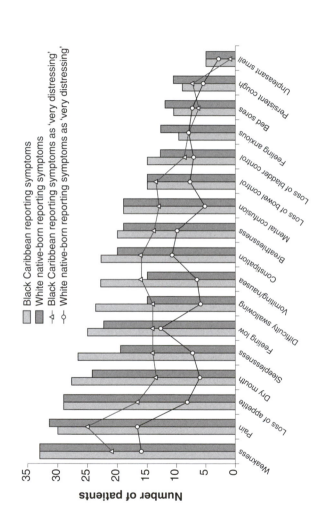

**Figure 15.1** Reported symptoms and symptom distress associated with advanced cancer (Black Caribbean n = 34, White n = 35). *Source*: Koffman J *et al*. Symptom severity and control of advanced cancer, assessed in two ethnic groups; interviews with bereaved family members and friends. *J Royal Soc Med*. 2003; 96: 10–16.

groups are more likely than the rest of the population to be poor.[40] Minority ethnic communities experience disadvantage – they are more likely to:

- live in deprived areas
- suffer all the problems that affect other people in these areas
- suffer the consequences of overt and inadvertent racial discrimination – individual and institutional.

---

**Self-assessment exercise 15.2**
**Time: 10 minutes**

The evidence strongly suggests that black and minority ethnic communities are under-represented in hospices.

- Why do you think this is so?
- What you would you suggest to improve uptake?

---

Allegations of poor access to healthcare services by black and minority ethnic groups are not new to the UK health service.[41,42] This is also an issue for end-of-life care where the impact of ageing on the black and minority ethnic groups now means larger numbers of older members within these communities will require health services for advanced disease.[7] A few reports have levelled criticism of care at the end of life for these communities and poor access to appropriate care. Low rates of cancer were seen as one explanation to account for low uptake of service provision, but the figures were likely to have been inaccurate because of inadequate ethnic monitoring.[43] One conclusion stated: *'some black and Asian patients and their carers are very disadvantaged, as they do not know what they are entitled to, and hence what to ask for by way of benefits and services'.*[44] A recent inner London health authority study demonstrated that black Caribbean patients with advanced disease experienced restricted access to some specialist palliative care services compared to white patients,[7] yet an analysis of local provision revealed no lack of palliative care services.[45] This example of under-utilisation of palliative care services by the black Caribbean community at the end of life supports other recent research among minority ethnic communities.[46,47] The explanations to account for this, all of which may operate in combination, are highlighted in Box 15.2.

## Communication issues among diverse communities

One of the main barriers to accessing specialist palliative care among black and *minority ethnic* communities is *communication*, with language problems being cited by patients, family members and professionals.[55] This has been shown to be a serious problem in GP consultations and causes misunderstandings.[56]

Other important communication difficulties arise where there is an over-reliance on the family acting on their loved one or dependant's behalf. While this may well be simpler than accessing an interpreter, it can potentially disadvantage the doctor and patient.[2] The family interpreter may filter, abbreviate or omit important information, or inform the doctor or the patient only what s/he thinks either needs

---

**Box 15.2 Black and minority ethnic social exclusion at the end of life: why does it occur?**

**Social deprivation**
Low socio-economic status has been positively linked to an increased likelihood of hospital deaths although this would apply equally to all population groups[48]

**Knowledge of specialist palliative care services and poor communication**
There is a growing body of evidence that black and ethnic minorities are not adequately aware of specialist palliative care services available to them.[50–52]

**Attitudes to palliative care**
Barriers to healthcare that the poor and the disenfranchised have traditionally encountered may affect their receptivity to palliative care.[49]

**Dissatisfaction with healthcare**
Uptake of health and social services among certain minority ethnic communities has revealed lower utilisation of services due to dissatisfaction with services.[53]

**Mistrust**
Evidence from USA to support the contention that black and minority ethnic groups are less likely than white patients to trust the motivations of doctors who discuss end-of-life care with them.[54]

**Ethno-centralism**
Demand for services may be influenced by the 'ethnocentric' outlook of palliative care services, discouraging black and minority ethnic groups from making use of relevant provision.[50]

**Gatekeepers**
Some healthcare professionals are 'gatekeepers' to services among minority ethnic groups, contributing to lower referral rates.[50]

---

to know. Important medical information may not be adequately understood or conveyed in full. Further, the use of children as interpreters is inappropriate. Details about an illness may be very intimate and it places an unfair burden on them, who, depending on their age, may be less likely to understand adult conversations in English, or for that matter even their own language. Using friends or untrained lay interpreters from the local community can be even more problematic since there can be issues of confidentiality and fear of gossip in the wider community.[57]

Communication may also involve:

- body language
- cultural rules as to what is courteous – e.g. not looking the professionals (especially the opposite gender) in the eye
- appropriate behaviours in an unequal gender and power relationship.[2]

People who speak English with a different accent or dialect may also be assumed to be less intelligent, or fail to be understood or understand what is being said to them.[57]

## The experience of informal caregivers from black and minority ethnic communities

The emphasis on care in the community rather than institutions, and the growing awareness that many more people would prefer to die at home given the choice,[58] means that informal caregivers are indispensable partners of the professional. Many assume responsibilities of care that were previously confined to specialist inpatient settings and community hospitals.[59] Caring for family members is regarded as an important obligation in the black Caribbean community.[60] Moreover, for many minority ethnic families, caring for dying relatives at home, when possible, is considered a matter of honour and integrity, as well as a means of ensuring the death occurs in a holy place.[61] Stigma, and loss of face, may result from not caring for close family.[6] In the Hindu tradition, the concepts of karma and sacred duty may place the family of a loved one or dependant under additional stress in order to do the right thing.[57] East London Bangladeshi children become actively involved in the care of a dying patient and in interactions with professionals, and act as interpreters.[61] This subsequently had a negative impact on them. A number of children were required to give up formal schooling, and older sons gave up work, to help with care of their dependants.

When there is home care, the burden often falls upon one person, but without ready access to outside support.[61] Multigenerational Pakistani and Bangladeshi families who wish to provide traditional support may also be in situations with high unemployment and poverty, and large families of young children.[62]

Home care is not without problems when outside help is needed, because many ethnic minorities would regard this as a sense of failure in the eyes of the community, and it may also be regarded as an invasion of privacy.[2] Tensions can arise when an elderly person needs and demands care from a female relative who may have quite different expectations, especially if the carer also has children born in Britain.[50] However, expectations of care from family relatives may change in coming years as patterns of family life and social networks evolve through a process of acculturation.

## Religious and spiritual issues at the end of life and during bereavement

The experience of advanced disease can have a profound effect on patients, family and friends. Indeed, during illness, many patients may raise questions that relate to their identity and self-worth as they seek to find the ultimate meaning in their life. Some patients attempt to answer these questions by examining their religious or spiritual beliefs. Formal religion is a means of expressing an underlying spirituality, but spiritual belief, concerned with the search for existential or the ultimate meaning in life, is a broader concept, and may not always be expressed in a religious way. This usually includes reference to a power other than self, often described as 'God', or 'forces of nature'.[63] This power is generally seen to help a person to transcend immediate experience and to re-establish hope. The importance of religion and spirituality among patients with advanced disease as a central component of physical and psychological wellbeing is increasingly recognised by professionals.[64] To this end, the acquisition of core competencies in the assessment and management of spiritual and religious care for specialist palliative care professionals has recently been highlighted.[65]

Most of the published literature on roles of religious faith at the end of life are descriptive and focus on 'fact-file' approaches to manage the experience of death and dying.[66–68] This approach is not without criticism as it has a tendency to over-categorise religious and cultural groups.[3]

---

**Self assessment exercise 15.3**
**Time: 10 minutes**

Religion and spirituality have been shown to offer support in times of crisis.

- What resources do you think are associated with them that might help patients with advanced disease and their families?

---

To date, little quantitative research has explored the presence and role of religious faith in helping patients with advanced disease and their families from black and minority ethnic communities living in the United Kingdom.[69] The few ethnographic studies that have explored the roles of religious faith have been limited to Asian communities and how they approach death and bereavement. One conducted in-depth research among the British Hindus living in Southampton.[57] Another has explored ageing and death among the Bangladeshi community living in Tower Hamlets in east London.[70] It has been argued that Laungani's contribution to understanding death and bereavement across cultures[71] demonstrates no evidence of ethnographic research of his own or wide ethnographic reading, and does not do justice to the diversity of Indian traditions.[2] There currently appears to be nothing at all on the black African or Chinese communities living and dying in the United Kingdom. This is clearly a major gap in the literature.

The lack of serious study of the religious and spiritual needs of minority ethnic communities may be partly due to an assumption that faith communities will provide their own religious and spiritual care. Anecdotal evidence from specialist palliative care nurses suggests that it is often assumed that ethnic minority patients have no spiritual problems because 'they have their own beliefs and rituals' – and, once again, 'they look after their own'.[2] While some models of palliative and supportive care have not included the role of spiritual care at the end of life, others have begun to acknowledge the important role of spirituality.[72] It has been suggested that lack of interest by professionals in patients' religious concerns may be due to the discomfort created by the discussion of personal matters, that they associate religion with 'superstition, intolerance and persecution', or that religion may be seen as a kind of consolation, a last resort, which is offered when all else fails.[73]

# Conclusion

The palliative care movement has assumed a leading role in addressing the health and social care needs of patients and families facing the inevitability of death. Yet it is only very recently that attention has focused on the importance of providing care for the increasingly diverse society in the United Kingdom. This has now become a demographic imperative. This chapter demonstrates that the language of understanding difference is complex yet fascinating. Further, when considering the influence of ethnicity and culture in the provision of care at the end of life, and during bereavement, we must endeavour to hold up two lenses, simultaneously. First, understanding and serving the needs of specific communities requires us to apply a framework of equity of provision. However, at the same time we must not lose sight of the individual and family before us, whose needs and concerns may not conform to our preconceived or stereotyped perceptions. *At the end of life, an individualised approach to care, with a focus on quality, is paramount for the patient – and family – regardless of his or her ethnic or cultural background.*

# References

1   World Health Organization. *National Cancer Control Programmes: policies and managerial guidelines*, 2nd edition. Geneva, World Health Organization; 2002.
2   Firth S. *Wider Horizons: care of the dying in a multi-cultural society*. London: National Council for Hospices and Specialist Palliative Care Services; 2001.
3   Gunaratnam Y. Culture is not enough. In: Field D, Hockey J, Small N, editors. *Death, Gender and Ethnicity*. London: Routledge; 2003, pp. 166–186.
4   Koffman J, Camps J. No way in: including the excluded at the end of life. In: Payne S, Seymour J, Skilbeck J *et al.*, editors. *Palliative Care Nursing: principles and evidence for practice*. Maidenhead: Open University Press; 2004.
5   Crawley L, Payne R, Bolden J *et al.* Palliative and end-of-life care in the African American community. *JAMA*. 2000; **284**: 2518–2521.
6   Karim K, Bailey M, Tunna K. Non white ethnicity and the provision of specialist palliative care services: factors affecting doctors' referral patterns *Pall Med*. 2000; **14**: 471–478.
7   Koffman J, Higginson IJ. Accounts of satisfaction with health care at the end of life: a comparison of first generation black Caribbeans and white patients with advanced disease. *Palliative Medicine*. 2001; **15**: 337–345.
8   Oliviere D. Culture and ethnicity. *Eur Jr Palliat Care*. 1999; **6**: 53–56.
9   Koffman J, Higginson IJ. A systematic review of race, ethnicity and culture as variables in palliative care research. *European Journal of Palliative Care*. 2005; 81.
10  Hillier S, Kelleher D. Considering culture, ethnicity and the politics of health. In: Hillier S, Kelleher D, editors. *Researching Cultural Differences in Health*. London: Routledge; 1996.
11  Gunaratnam Y. *Researching 'Race' and Ethnicity: methods, knowledge and power*. London: Sage; 2003.
12  Collins. *Collins Concise Dictionary*. Glasgow: HarperCollins Publishers; 2001.
13  Stepan N. *The Idea of Race in Science*. London: MacMillan Press; 1982.
14  Gould SJ. *The Mismeasure of Man*. Harmondsworth: Penguin; 1981.
15  Singh SP. Ethnicity in psychiatric epidemiology: need for precision. *British Journal of Psychiatry*. 1997; **171**: 305–308.
16  Ahmad WIU. *'Race' and Health in Contemporary Britain*. London: Open University Press; 1993.
17  Karlesen S, Nazroo JY. Relation between discrimination, social class and health among ethnic minority groups. *American Journal of Public Health*. 2002; **92**(4): 624–631.
18  Chaturvedi N. Ethnicity as an epidemiological determinant – crude racist or crucially important? *International Journal of Epidemiology*. 2001; **30**: 925–927.
19  Afshari R, Bhopal RS. Changing pattern of the use of 'ethnicity' and 'race' in scientific literature. *International Journal of Epidemiology*. 2002; **31**: 1074–1076.

20 Senior A, Bhopal R. Ethnicity as a variable in epidemiological research. *BMJ*. 1994; **309**: 327–330.

21 DeGiovanni JK, Beevers DG, Jackson SHD *et al*. The Birmingham blood pressure school study. *Postgraduate Medical Journal*. 1983; **59**: 627–629.

22 Barker RM, Baker MR. Incidence of cancer in Bradford Asians. *Journal of Epidemiology and Community Health*. 1990; **44**: 125–129.

23 Coleman D. Ethnic intermarriage in Great Britain. *Population Trends*. 1985; **40**: 4–10.

24 Koffman J, Higginson IJ. Minority ethnic groups and our healthier nation. *Journal of Public Health Medicine*. 2000; **22**(2): 245.

25 Cruikshank JK, Beevers DG. Migration, ethnicity, health and disease. In: Cruikshank JK, Beevers DG, editors. *Ethnic Factors in Health and Disease*. London: Wright; 1989.

26 Bhopal RS. *Ethnicity, Race, Health and Research: racist, black box, junk or enlightened epidemiology?* University of Newcastle: Department of Epidemiology and Public Health; 1995.

27 Pringle M, Rothera I. *Ethnic Group Data Collection in Primary Care: problems and solutions*. Nottingham, University of Nottingham Medical School; 1995.

28 Bhopal RS, Phillimore P, Kohli HS. Inappropriate use of the term 'Asian': an obstacle to ethnicity and health research. *Journal of Public Health Medicine*. 1991; **13**: 244–246

29 Department of Health. *Inequalities in Health: report of an independent inquiry chaired by Sir Donald Acheson*. London: The Stationery Office; 1998.

30 Mechanic D. *Medical Sociology*. New York: Free Press; 1978.

31 Donovan J. *We Don't Buy Sickness, It Just Comes*. Aldershot: Gower; 1986.

32 Hofstede G. *Cultures and Organisations - software of the mind*. London: Profile Business; 1991.

33 Helman C. *Culture, Health and Illness*, 4th edition. Oxford: Butterworth-Heinemann; 2000.

34 McKenzie KJ, Crowcroft NS. Race, ethnicity, culture and science. *British Medical Journal*. 1994; **309**: 286–287.

35 Zborowski M. Cultural components in response to pain. *Journal of Society Issues*. 1952; **8**: 16–30.

36 Koffman J, Higginson IJ, Donaldson N. Symptom severity in advanced cancer assessed in two ethnic groups by interviews with bereaved family members and friends. *Journal of the Royal Society of Medicine*. 2003; **96**: 10–16.

37 Lasch KE. Culture and pain. *Pain Clinical Updates*. December 2002; **10**(5).

38 Krause I. The sinking heart, a Punjabi communication of distress. *Soc Sci Med*. 2005; **29**(4): 563–575.

39 Ahmed T. The Asian experience. In: Salman R, Bahal V, editors. *Assessing Health Needs in People from Minority Ethnic Groups*. London: Royal College of Physicians; 1998.

40 Berthoud R, Modood T. Ethnic minorities in Britain: diversity and disadvantage. In: Berthoud R, editor. *The Fourth National Survey of Ethnic Minorities*. London: Policy Studies Institute; 1997, pp. 159–160.

41 O'Neill J, Marconi K. Access to palliative care in the USA: why emphasize vulnerable populations? *J R Soc Med*. 2001; **94**: 452–454.

42 Harding S, Maxwell R. Difference in mortality of migrants. In: Drever F, Whitehead M, editors. *Health Inequalities: decennial supplement series DS no. 15*. London: The Stationery Office; 1997.

43 Aspinall PJ. Ethnic groups and our healthier nation: whither the information base? *Journal of Public Health Medicine*. 1999; **21**: 125–132.

44 Hill D, Penso D. *Opening Doors: improving access to hospice and specialist palliative care services by members of the black and ethnic minority communities*. Occasional Paper 7. London: National Council for Hospice and Specialist Palliative Care Services; 1995.

45 Eve A, Smith AM, Tebbit P. Hospice and palliative care in the UK 1994–5, including a summary of trends 1990–5. *Palliat Med*. 1997; **11**(1): 31–43.

46 Farrell J. *Do Disadvantaged and Minority Ethnic Groups Receive Adequate Access to Palliative Care Services?* Glasgow: Glasgow University; 2000.

47 Skilbeck J, Corner J, Leech N *et al*. Clinical nurse specialists in palliative care. Part 1. A description of the Macmillan nurse caseload. *Palliat Med*. 2002; **16**(4): 285–296.

48 Higginson IJ, Webb D, Lessof L. Reducing hospital beds for patients with advanced cancer. *The Lancet*. 1994; **344**(8919): 409.

49 Gibson R. Palliative care for the poor and disenfranchised: a view from the Robert Wood Johnson Foundation. *J R Soc Med*. 2001; **94**: 486–489.

50  Smaje C, Field D. Absent minorities? Ethnicity and the use of palliative care services. In: Hockey J, Small N, editors. *Death, Gender and Ethnicity*. London: Routledge; 1997. pp. 142–165.

51  Kurent JE. Beyond ethnicity [comment]. *Journal of Pain and Symptom Management*. 2003; **25**(2): 194–195.

52  Harron-Iqbal H, Field D, Parker H *et al*. Palliative care services in Leicester. *International Journal of Palliative Nursing*. 1995; **1**: 114–116.

53  Lindsay J, Jagger C, Hibbert M *et al*. Knowledge, uptake and the availability of health and social services among Asian Gujarati and white persons. *Ethnicity and Health*. 1997; **2**: 59–69.

54  Caralis PV, Davis B, Wright K *et al*. The influence of ethnicity and race on attitudes toward advanced directives, life-prolonging treatments, and euthanasia. *Journal of Clinical Ethics*. 1993; **4**: 155–165.

55  Nazroo JY. *Ethnicity and Mental Health*. London: Policy Studies Institute; 1997.

56  Koffman J, Higginson IJ. Accounts of carers' satisfaction with health care at the end of life: a comparison of first generation black Caribbeans and white patients with advanced disease. *Palliative Medicine*. 2001; **15**(4): 337–345.

57  Firth S. *Dying, Death and Bereavement in the British Hindu Community*. Leuven: Peeters; 1997.

58  Gomes B, Higginson IJ. Home or hospital: choices at the end of life. *J R Soc Med*. 2004; **97**(9): 413–414.

59  Rhodes P, Shaw S. Informal care and terminal illness. *Health and Social Care in the Community*. 1999; **7**: 39–50.

60  Koffman J, Higginson IJ. Fit to care? A comparison of informal caregivers of first generation black Caribbeans and white dependants with advanced progressive disease in the United Kingdom. *Health and Social Care in the Community*. 2003; **11**(6): 528–536.

61  Spruyt O. Community-based palliative care for Bangladeshi patients in east London: accounts of bereaved carers. *Palliative Medicine*. 1999; **13**: 119–129.

62  Blakemore K. Health and social care needs in minority communities: an over problemitized issue? *Health and Social Care in the Community*. 2000; **8**(1): 22–30.

63  Speck P. Spiritual issues in palliative care. In: Doyle D, Hanks GWC, MacDonald N, editors. *Oxford Textbook of Palliative Care*. Oxford: Oxford University Press; 1998, pp. 805–814.

64  Kearney M, Mount B. Spiritual care of the dying patient. In: Chochinov H, Breitbart W, editors. *Handbook of Psychiatry in Palliative Care*. New York: Oxford University Press; 2000, pp. 357–393.

65  National Institute for Clinical Excellence. *Guidance on Cancer Services: improving supportive and palliative care for adults with cancer*. London: National Institute for Clinical Excellence; 2004.

66  Neuberger J. *Caring for Dying People of Different Faiths*. Oxford: Radcliffe Medical Press; 2004.

67  Katz JS. Jewish perspectives on death, dying and bereavement. In: Dickerson D, Johnson M, editors. *Death, Dying and Bereavement*. London: Sage Publications; 2001, p. 207.

68  Koffman J. Rituals surrounding death and dying within the black Caribbean community. *Palliative Care Today*. 2001; **10**: 7.

69  Koffman J, Higginson IJ. Religious faith and support at the end of life: a comparison of first generation black Caribbean and white populations. *Palliative Medicine*. 2002; **16**(6): 540–541.

70  Gardner K. Death, burial and bereavement amongst Bengali Muslims. *Journal of Ethnic and Migration Studies*. 1998; **24**(3): 507–521.

71  Laungani P. Death in a Hindu family. In: Parkes CM, Laungani P, Young B, editors. *Death and Bereavement Across Cultures*. Hove: Brunner Routledge; 2000, pp. 52–72.

72  Ellershaw J, Smith C, Overhill S *et al*. Care of the dying: setting standards for symptom control in the last 48 hours of life. *Journal of Pain and Symptom Management*. 2001; **21**: 12–17.

73  Dein S, Stygall J. Does being religious help or hinder coping with chronic illness? A critical literature review. *Palliative Medicine*. 1997; **11**(4): 291–298.

# To learn more

- Firth S. *Wider Horizons: care of the dying in a multi-cultural society*. London: National Council for Hospices and Specialist Palliative Care Services; 2001.
- Gunarantnam Y. *Researching 'Race' and Ethnicity': methods, knowledge and power*. London: Sage; 2003.

- Koffman J, Camps J. No way in: including the excluded at the end of life. In: Payne S, Seymour J, Skilbeck J *et al.*, editors. *Palliative Care Nursing: principles and evidence for practice.* Maidenhead: Open University Press; 2004.
- Murray Parkes C, Laugani P *et al. Death and Bereavement Across Cultures.* Hove: Brunner-Routledge; 2003.
- Neuberger J. *Caring for Dying People of Different Faiths.* Oxford: Radcliffe Medical Press; 2004.
- Purnell LD, Paulanka BJ. *Transcultural Health Care: a culturally competent approach,* 2nd edition. Philadelphia: FA Davis Company; 2003.

# Complementary chapters

*See also Stepping into Palliative Care 1: relationships and responses*

- Chapter 2: What is palliative care?
- Chapter 4: The experience of illness
- Chapter 5: The psychological impact of serious illness
- Chapter 6: Hope and coping strategies
- Chapter 16: Sexuality and palliative care

*See also Stepping into Palliative Care 2: care and practice*

- Chapter 1: Assessment in palliative care
- Chapter 11: Breaking bad news
- Chapter 12: Hearing the pain of the carer
- Chapter 13: Spirituality and palliative care
- Chapter 14: Bereavement

# Chapter 16

# Sexuality and palliative care

*Jon Hibberd*

---

**Pre-reading exercise 16.1**
**Time: 15 minutes**

Before reading this chapter, reflect on your understanding of sexuality.

- What impact does it have upon you?
- How do you see it expressed?
- Are you comfortable in raising the subject with patients?

---

## Introduction

The chapter objectives are:

- to explore definitions of sexuality in the context of palliative care
- to explore expressions of sexuality in the context of palliative care
- to address the 'taboo factor', and to help professionals overcome difficulties in addressing the issue of sexuality with patients
- to present examples of best practice.

## Defining sexuality

Numerous attempts have been made to define sexuality with differing emphasis placed on its social, psychological, spiritual and physical attributes. The fact that so many definitions exist suggests that, as an integral component of who each person is, it is unique. Sexuality is key to our self-understanding and social role but it is also a private, hidden aspect of ourselves that we may choose, or not choose, to share with others.[1]

Sexuality comes into all aspects of existence, involving biological and social aspects of the body. It is complex and contextual.[2]

If the definitions are placed within the context of palliation, their importance becomes vital in the care of patients with cancer and other life-threatening disorders. Such conditions have a significant physical, emotional, social and spiritual effect upon all aspects of a person's sexuality. In all its diversity, it is inevitably affected.

---

**Self-assessment exercise 16.1**
**Time: 15 minutes**

For someone experiencing cancer or other life-threatening disorder, how do you think his or her sexuality will be affected?
  Try to group your thoughts into headings, e.g.:

- *physical* – change in body image and weight loss
- *emotional* – anxiety, fear, low self-esteem and anger
- *social* – touch, communication and impact on work
- *spiritual* – challenge to faith, finding a spiritual faith/path.

---

When answering Self-assessment exercise 16.1 you will have identified many examples that illustrate clearly how important sexuality is in our lives. It is fundamental to the way people:

- share intimacy
- experience physical closeness
- view themselves
- are perceived by others.

Sexuality and body image are closely linked with roles and relationships within families, at work and in society.[3] It includes, but should never be limited to, sexual intercourse and sexual function.

## Expressing sexuality

A way of looking at sexuality is demonstrated in *the sexuality flower model* (Figure 16.1).

---

**Self-assessment exercise 16.2**
**Time: 15 minutes**

Look at *the sexuality flower model* (Figure 16.1), then reflect on:

- what you have done today
- the emotions and feelings you have experienced
- the communication you have had with adults, children; even animals.

---

You should be able to identify many words in *the sexuality flower model* that would describe what you have experienced. Possibly, several words would describe your experience, embracing an action accompanied by an emotion or feeling. *This is your unique, personal expression of sexuality.*

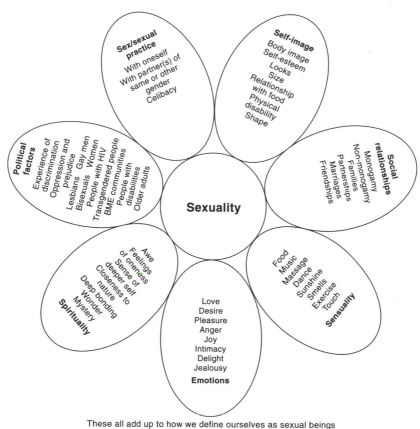

These all add up to how we define ourselves as sexual beings
Sexuality = sexual self-hood
Sexuality involves our relationships with ourselves, those around us and the society in which we
live — whether we identify as heterosexual, gay, lesbian, bisexual or celibate

**Figure 16.1**  The sexuality flower model.*

## Case scenarios

Each of the following four case scenarios illustrates an expression of sexuality. They are all real experiences. Names have been changed to protect identities.

---

**Case scenario 16.1**

Scott was in the terminal phase of acquired immune deficiency syndrome (AIDS) in the bedded unit of a hospice. Paul visited daily, and as Scott's condition worsened, Paul stayed for longer periods. The staff on the unit encouraged Paul to become involved in the personal care of Scott; something that Paul and Scott always shared when Scott was at home.

---

\* Permission was kindly given to use this model by Carol Painter and Jo Adams of the Centre for HIV and Sexual Health in Sheffield. Model originally used in their training manual *Sexuality: Explore, Dream, Discover* (2004). For more information: tel: 0114 261 900; email: admin@chiv.nhs.uk

> It was one morning while Paul and Scott were alone together in the room, while Paul was washing Scott, that Scott died peacefully in Paul's arms. Paul said after that in that intimate moment they shared together it felt as though they had been enfolded in a blanket of peace and love. A very sacred moment.

In Case scenario 16.1, sexuality was expressed through:

- gay partnership
- touch
- love
- intimacy
- feelings of oneness
- spirituality
- body image.

---

**Case scenario 16.2**

Muriel was in the final stages of lung cancer, being cared for at home by Frank, her husband, and their large family of three daughters and grandchildren. The family came from the East End of London. They were a vibrant, colourful, united family of whom Muriel was clearly the head.

Muriel and Frank throughout their married life always took their afternoon rest together when possible; they continued with this routine right up until Muriel's death. Muriel died peacefully at home. Frank said that Muriel and he had had a very close relationship.

---

In Case scenario 16.2, sexuality was expressed through:

- heterosexual partnership
- marriage
- sexual practice with partner
- touch
- love
- intimacy.

---

**Case scenario 16.3**

Gemma and Helen had not long moved following early retirement. Gemma, prior to moving, had been diagnosed with endometrial cancer. In spite of the diagnosis, they went ahead with their planned relocation.

Gemma and Helen shared a long-term relationship together, and enjoyed a very active life, walking, cycling, rock climbing, etc. These activities were curtailed as Gemma's health deteriorated.

Gemma was very much in touch with her mortality and shared her feelings openly. She and Helen spoke about their relationship, that it was based upon love, trust and openness between each other. Gemma said that she wished her funeral to be a celebration of love and its expression in many forms.

In Case scenario 16.3, sexuality was expressed through:

- lesbian partnership
- physical disability
- exercise
- pleasure
- love
- closeness to nature
- sense of deeper self.

---

**Case scenario 16.4**

Gina and Tom had been married for 62 years; both were in their mid-eighties. Tom had become unwell over several months and was eventually admitted to hospital with obstructive jaundice. Cancer of the pancreas was diagnosed.

While Tom was in hospital, Gina suffered a massive heart attack at home and died on arrival at the hospital where Tom was a patient. Their son broke the news to Tom of his wife's sudden death.

Tom died 6 weeks after Gina, in a nursing home. In the hours leading up to his death, the nursing staff stayed with him and reported afterwards that he spoke for a long time about the good life he had shared with Gina over the years.

The card Tom wrote for his floral tribute at Gina's funeral read:

*'To my dearest Gina. Be with you very soon my darling. Your Tommy.'*

---

In Case scenario 16.4, sexuality was expressed through:

- heterosexual partnership
- marriage
- friendship
- memories
- love
- intimacy
- bonding
- older age.

Each case scenario, different and profound. The people in them were different and expressed their unique characteristics of sexuality.

# Addressing the 'taboo'

Until now, the focus has been about raising awareness of the influence of sexuality. This section takes a different approach in attempting to dispel the fears that many professionals have in addressing the subject of sexuality with patients and the family.

The main difficulty that professionals experience is *'I don't know what to say.'* This can be for many reasons, which we will touch upon later. Sexuality exists separately from sexual function.[4] Often, the two terms are used synonymously. However, confusion often arises because they are different aspects of the same complex of emotions and behaviours.

---

**Self-assessment exercise 16.3**
**Time: 15 minutes**

- *Think* – about your understanding of the difference between sexuality and sexual function.
- *Reflect* – on these issues and their impact on you.

---

Patients may wish to talk about the difficulties they are experiencing with their sexuality or sexual function. However, they may not know *how* to talk about it or *who* to talk to. It is important not to assume that a patient, who does not initiate discussion, does not have concerns about sexuality. Patients often *'suffer in silence'* because they assume that if sexuality and intimacy were important, professionals would discuss them.[5]

As individuals, and professionals, we have our own unique set of beliefs, attitudes and values. These influence whether we perceive issues of sexuality to be an integral part of patient care.

---

**Self-assessment exercise 16.4**
**Time: 20 minutes**

This exercise is challenging. Listed are reasons why professionals feel unable to address sexuality.
1 *Reflect on these.*
2 *Which influences your approach?*

- I don't know what to say.
- I don't think sexuality is an issue for patients with cancer.
- My religious belief inhibits me from talking of such things.
- I need special training to talk about something so personal with patients.
- I would feel very embarrassed about talking about it.
- It just never enters my mind to talk about it with patients.
- That's someone else's job to deal with that sort of thing.
- I think it's a vital part of patient care. I do address the issue of sexuality.

---

It could be that you did not identify with any of the comments in Self-assessment exercise 16.4. Nurses still need to learn about:

- the professional use of self
- having a high level of self-knowledge
- the uniqueness and value of others.[6]

> **Self-assessment exercise 16.5**
> **Time: 15 minutes**
>
> Look at *the sexuality flower model* (Figure 16.1 on page 189).
>
> • How well do you know yourself?

Being comfortable with one's sexual identity, and all that embraces, is important when working with patients. You have a key role to play in helping patients and family resolve difficulties they may be experiencing with their sexuality. People with advanced disease have little time and may often feel robbed of past joys, which their sexuality may help them to regain.[3]

# Examples of best practice

Here we look at three case scenarios using key skills in communication, which may help you feel confident in addressing the issue of sexuality with patients and family.

*Before reading on, reflect on the following seven points.*[7,8] This list was devised as prerequisites for addressing needs relating to a patient's sexuality.

1 *Assessment and timing* – ongoing assessment and appropriate timing of discussion.
2 *Self-awareness of the interviewer* – acknowledge own prejudice and bias; be willing to put these to one side.
3 *Privacy* – setting and timing.
4 *Confidentiality* – acknowledge confidentiality with patient.
5 *Permission giving* – gain patient's permission to talk or not.
6 *Language* – use appropriate language.
7 *Boundaries* – set time boundaries for self and patient.

> **Case scenario 16.5**
>
> Annie and Grace have been in a relationship living together for 15 years. Both women had been in heterosexual relationships before they met and each have children all in their late twenties and early thirties from these previous relationships.
>
> Grace has cancer of the lung and is gradually becoming more reliant on Annie for help.

## Identified problems

• Grace feels she is losing her identity as a mother. Both her daughters are expecting babies within the next 6 months. Grace feels she wants some involvement in planning for the birth of her new grandchildren, but feels time is running out.
• Grace feels she is not fulfilling her physical sexual role with Annie. Annie is desperate to reassure and help Grace but does not know how.

- Due to the cancer, the effect on Grace's body image is beginning to show. Grace has lost a lot of weight and Grace no longer feels attractive, particularly for Annie.

## Suggested interventions

- Use open-ended questioning to ascertain Grace and Annie's understanding and concerns, e.g.:
  - How do you wish to be involved in the planning of the birth of your grandchildren?
  - Many people with cancer experience difficulties with the physical/sexual side of their relationship because of the symptoms. What is causing you the most problem?
- Suggest Grace starts to compile a memory box, filling it with small gifts, mementoes, photographs, letters and heirlooms that her grandchildren would have after Grace has died.
- Grace identifies that fatigue and breathlessness affect her lovemaking with Annie. Suggest they identify the best time of day when Grace has more energy, less pain, few problems with breathing. Encourage them to explore with each other what they enjoy sharing together physically that does not cause Grace distress. Suggest touch, stroking, gentle massage, holding and caressing.
- Suggest taking breakthrough analgesia before times of intimacy.
- Encourage Grace and Annie to prioritise ways in which Grace can feel better about her body image. What gives her most pleasure? What does she like wearing? How does she like her hair styled? Does she wear jewellery? Encourage Grace to look upon each day as her day and to reward herself with at least one treat each day that makes her feel good about herself.
- Discuss with Grace and the medical team the most appropriate use of steroids to help elevate Grace's mood and increase body weight by stimulating her appetite.
- Review situation every 7 to 10 days.
- Seek advice from other members of the multidisciplinary team if you are unsure of how to help or what to say.
- Bring issues of concern to your clinical supervision.

---

**Case scenario 16.6**

Mike and Doreen are in their mid-sixties, having been married for over 30 years. Mike has been diagnosed with cancer of the oesophagus and has been undergoing a trial of chemotherapy treatment.

---

## Identified problems

- Mike and Doreen have always been active sexually together, but due to Mike's illness he is very fatigued and cannot sustain an erection.
- Doreen is at a loss on how she can help make things easier for Mike. Mike feels that he is not fulfilling his role as husband.
- Mike and Doreen find it difficult to discuss the subject because they feel embarrassed about talking on such an intimate matter.

## Suggested interventions

- Give reassurance. Explain that the difficulty Mike is experiencing is common with men who have cancer.
- Suggest non-penetrative sexual activity such as mutual massage, caressing, rubbing, and holding each other. Suggest buying or borrowing from the library a book on sexual health where it illustrates alternative positioning for sexual intercourse.
- Encourage Mike to identify the times of day when he feels less fatigued and he could sustain sexual activity.
- Suggest to Mike and Doreen that some medication to help address Mike's erectile dysfunction may help. Offer to liaise with the GP on their behalf or request a visit by the GP so that Mike and Doreen can discuss things in private.
- Review situation every 7 to 10 days.
- Reflect and be aware of any difficulties you may have in dealing with this situation. Is there anything you need to bring to clinical supervision?

---

### Case scenario 16.7

Trudy and Roger are in their early forties. They have been married for over 20 years and have three teenage children. Trudy has a recurrence of her breast cancer with liver secondaries. She has commenced an aggressive regime of chemotherapy, which is taking its toll on Trudy physically. Roger is finding it difficult to cope emotionally.

---

## Identified problems

- Roger admits he does not know how to get close to Trudy physically any more. He feels she is pushing him away.
- The teenage children sense tension in the home and are finding things difficult.

## Suggested interventions

- Encourage Roger to identify and verbalise his specific difficulties by using open reflective questions, e.g. *'You spoke earlier of the physical difficulties you are having. Can you be more specific about these so I can understand more clearly what's going on for you and Trudy?'*
- Suggest a meeting with Trudy, facilitated by you, and encourage Roger to verbalise to Trudy how he is feeling.
- Use empathic verbal interventions/questions with Trudy, e.g. *'I can see this treatment is really taking its toll on you physically. Can Roger help in any way to make things easier for you?'*
- In the light of Roger's verbalised feeling, seek to elicit a response from Trudy again through open questions, e.g. *'What do you feel about what Roger has said?'*; *'Do you want to talk about this now?'*
- This situation is potentially extremely sensitive, particularly as there are teenagers involved. It could be that you need to bring these issues to the wider multidisciplinary team, e.g. clinical nurse specialist in palliative care, hospice family support workers, who have expertise on how to deal with such situations.

- Always seek the permission of Trudy and Roger to get external advice if you are experiencing difficulty in providing the answers.
- Do not feel guilty that you do not have all the answers.
- Think 'teamwork'. Is there anyone else who can help with these problems?
- Be aware of yourself, your own emotions and feelings.
- Consider 'debriefing' after a session so that you do not emotionally hold their projected feelings.

In these three case scenarios, differing interventions have been used to help people address their sexual difficulties. Problems with sexuality and sexual function can often have a 'spin-off' effect, e.g. exacerbating feelings of low self-esteem and low self-worth. These feelings, if not addressed, may cause difficulties in relationship that assume greater magnitude than they are.

Each situation you encounter will be different. Therefore, it is important to remember the five basic principles that hold true for any situation:

1 active listening
2 reflecting back to check thoughts and feelings
3 be empathic
4 do not judge
5 be self-aware.

The four misconceptions held are:

1 *age* – do not assume that sexuality and sexual function is no longer important to individuals of mature years
2 *heterosexuality* – do not ignore the possibility of homosexual/lesbian relationships
3 *being single* – do not assume that sexuality and sexual function is not an issue for people not in a relationship
4 *palliative care status* – do not assume that patients in the advanced stage of disease have no interest in sexual activity.

## Conclusion

This chapter aimed to raise awareness of sexuality and sexual function. Hopefully, it has offered some guidelines on how to approach this sensitive subject. The aim has been to help you to:

- recognise the importance of sexuality
- listen to patients' concerns
- assess a situation and always review it
- help to create a space for sexuality to be expressed and maintained
- respect and support self-image
- maintain a person's dignity
- use the expertise of the wider team.

Harvey Milk,[10] an American campaigner for sexual equality, said:

*If we are not free to be ourselves in that most human of all activities, the expression of love, then life itself loses its meaning!*

# References

1 Cox K. Sexual identity – gender and sexual orientation. In: Oliviere D, Monroe B, editors. *Death, Dying and Social Differences*. Oxford: Oxford University Press; 2004.
2 Lawler J. *Behind the Screens*. Melbourne: Churchill Livingstone; 1991.
3 Rice AM. Sexuality in cancer and palliative care 1: effects on disease and treatment. *Int J of Palliative Nursing*. 2000; **6**(8): 392–397.
4 Shell JA, Smith CK. Sexuality and the older person with cancer. *Oncology Nurses Forum*. 1994; **21**: 553–558.
5 Hughes MK. Sexuality and the cancer survivor. *Cancer Nursing*. 2000; **23**: 477–482.
6 Antrobus S. Developing the nurse as a knowledge worker in health: learning the artistry of practice. *Journal of Advanced Nursing*. 1997; **25**: 829–835.
7 Dittemar S, editor. *Rehabilitation Nursing*. New York: Mosby; 1989.
8 Fogel CI, Lawer D. *Sexual Health Promotion*. Philadelphia: WB Saunders Co; 1990.
9 White K. Sexuality and body image. In: O'Connor M, Aranda S, editors. *Palliative Care Nursing: a guide to practice*. Oxford: Radcliffe Medical Press; 2003.
10 Shilts R. *The Mayor of Castro Street: the life and times of Harvey Milk*. New York: St Martin's Press; 1982.

# To learn more

• Champion A. Male cancer and sexual function. *Sexual and Marital Therapy II*. 1996; **11**(3): 227–244.
• Fallowfield L. The quality of life: sexual function and body image following cancer therapy. *Cancer Topics*. 1992; **9**: 20–21.
• Maguire P, Faulkner A, Booth K *et al.* Helping cancer patients disclose their concerns. *European Journal of Cancer – A*. 1996; **32**(1): 78–81.
• Nazarko I, Aylott J, Andrews A. Dilemmas: how should nurses respond to patients' sexual needs? *Nursing Times*. 2000; **96**(5): 35.
• Price B. A model for body image care. *Journal of Advanced Nursing*. 1990; **15**(5): 585–593.
• Roper N, Logan WW, Tierney AJ. *The Elements of Nursing*, 2nd edition. Edinburgh: Churchill Livingstone; 1990.
• Schover LR. *Better Sex After Serious Illness*. Bottom Line/Health. 2002: 16(6): 11–13.
• Stead ML, Fallowfield L, Brown JM *et al.* Communication about sexual problems and sexual concerns in ovarian cancer: qualitative study. *BMJ*. 2001; **323**: 836–837.
• Webb C. Nurses' knowledge and attitudes about sexuality in health care. *Int J of Nursing Studies*. 1987; **25**(3): 235–244.

# Complementary chapters

*See also Stepping into Palliative Care 1: relationships and responses*

• Chapter 3: The cancer journey
• Chapter 4: The experience of illness
• Chapter 5: The psychological impact of serious illness

*See also Stepping into Palliative Care 2: care and practice*

• Chapter 13: Spirituality and palliative care

# Useful contacts

**Alzheimer's Disease Society**
Gordon House, 10 Greencoat Place, London SW1P 1PH
General enquiries: 020 7306 0606
Helpline: 08453 000 336 (8:30 am to 6:30 pm, Monday to Friday)
Email: info@alzheimers.org.uk
Website: www.alzheimers.org.uk

The Alzheimer's Disease Society is a care and research charity for people with Alzheimer's disease and other forms of dementia, their families and carers. It is a national membership organisation and works through nearly 300 branches and support groups. There is a wealth of information available on the website including fact and advice sheets.

**Bereavement Research Forum**
Bereavement Research Forum Administrator, Bereavement Service
St Joseph's Hospice, Mare Street, Hackney, London E8 4SA
Tel: 020 8525 6031
Email: s.cornford@stjh.org.uk
Website: www.brforum.org.uk

The Bereavement Research Forum provides opportunities for the discussion and development of bereavement research and the promotion of research into policy and practice. Three symposia are held annually and a conference every other year. The website gives further information about the organisation, membership and activities.

**Breast Cancer Care**
Kiln House, 210 New Kings Road, London SW6 4NZ
Tel: 020 7384 2984
Helpline: 0808 800 6000 (9 am to 5 pm, Monday to Friday; 9 am to 2 pm, Saturday)
Fax: 020 7384 3387
Email: info@breastcancercare.org.uk
Website: www.breastcancercare.org.uk

Breast Cancer Care offers practical advice, information and support to women concerned about breast cancer. Its services include a wide range of booklets, leaflets and audiotapes, a prosthesis-fitting service and one-to-one emotional support from volunteers who have experienced breast cancer. BCC aims to help anyone who needs its services – women with breast cancer, with other breast-related problems or who are worried about their breast health, families, partners and friends, members of the general public who need information, doctors, nurses and other health professionals, and the media.

### Bristol Cancer Help Centre
Grove House, Cornwallis Grove, Bristol BS8 4PG
Reception: 01179 809 500
Helpline: 08451 232 310 (9:30 am to 5 pm weekdays or 24-hour answerphone)
Email: info@bristolcancerhelp.org ; Helpline@bristolcancerhelp.org
Website: www.bristolcancerhelp.org

Bristol Cancer Help Centre is the holistic charity that pioneered the *Bristol Approach* to cancer care, for people with cancer and those close to them. The Bristol Approach works hand in hand with medical treatment, providing a unique combination of physical, emotional and spiritual support, using complementary therapies and self-help techniques, including practical advice on nutrition. People can access the Bristol Approach through residential courses run by experienced teams of doctors, nurses and complementary therapists.

### British Heart Foundation
14 Fitzhardinge Street, London W1H 6DH
Tel: 020 7935 0185
Email: bhfnurses@bhf.org.uk
Website: www.bhf.org.uk

Every 2 minutes, heart and circulatory disease kills one person in the UK. It can strike anyone at any time. Voluntary donations have helped the British Heart Foundation make tremendous advances in the diagnosis, treatment and prevention of heart and circulatory disease. However, it remains our biggest killer.

### CancerBACUP
3 Bath Place, Rivington Street, London EC2A 3JR
United Kingdom
Tel: 020 7696 9003
Fax: 020 7696 9002
Cancer information helpline (UK only): 0808 800 1234 (lines staffed by cancer specialist nurses, 9 am to 8 pm, Monday to Friday)
Email: info@cancerbacup.org
Website: www.cancerbacup.org

CancerBACUP offers a free cancer information service staffed by qualified and experienced cancer nurses, and publications on all aspects of cancer written specifically for patients and their families (available in full on the website) and a growing number of CancerBACUP local centres in hospitals staffed by specialist cancer nurses. The nurses are supported by around 200 cancer specialists to help them provide the highest quality information. The database holds a comprehensive list of resources, organisations and support groups for cancer patients. CancerBACUP supports health professionals with information on controversial and difficult cancer topics written specifically for doctors and with the most comprehensive listing of UK cancer treatment guidelines.

**CancerHelp UK**
Website: www.cancerhelp.org.uk
*CancerHelp UK can only give information on the internet*

CancerHelp UK is a free information service (provided by Cancer Research UK) about cancer and cancer care for people with cancer and their families. They believe that information about cancer should be freely available to all and written in a way that people can easily understand.

**Cancer Research UK**
PO Box 123, Lincoln's Inn Fields, London WC2A 3PX
Tel (Supporter Services): 020 7121 6699
Tel (Switchboard): 020 7242 0200
Fax: 020 7269 3100
Email: supporter.services@cancer.org.uk
Website: www.cancerresearchuk.org

Cancer Research UK is dedicated to research on the causes, treatment and prevention of cancer. Their vision is to conquer cancer through world-class research, aiming to control the disease within two generations. They support the work of over 3000 scientists, doctors and nurses working across the UK. Their annual scientific spend is more than £213 million, which is raised almost entirely through public donations.

**Carers National Association**
20/25 Glasshouse Yard, London EC1A 4JT
Tel: 020 7490 8818
Fax: 020 7490 8824
Tel (Carersline – advice line for carers): 0345 573 369
Website: www.londonhealth.co.uk/carersnationalassociation.asp

The Carers National Association is the national voice of carers in the UK. Their work involves:

- raising awareness at all levels of government and society of the needs of carers and ensuring action is taken to support them
- helping carers become more aware of their own role and status in the community
- providing information, advice and support to carers, enabling them to make their own choices about providing care
- cooperation with primary healthcare teams, helping them to recognise and support carers in their surgeries
- believing that carers who want to continue in paid work should be encouraged to do so; they offer companies advice and training on developing carer-friendly policies
- pressing for guaranteed respite breaks for carers, at times that are right for the carer and the person they care for.

## The Compassionate Friends
53 North Street, Bristol BS3 1EN
Tel: 08451 203 785
Fax: 08451 203 786
Helpline: 08451 232 304 (10 am to 4 pm, 6:30 pm to 10:30 pm,
open every day of the year)
Email: info@tcf.org.uk
Website: www.tcf.org.uk

The Compassionate Friends is an organisation of bereaved parents and their families offering understanding, support and encouragement to others after the death of a child or children. They also offer support, advice and information to other relatives, friends and professionals who are helping the family. The helpline is answered by a bereaved parent who is there to listen when you need someone to talk to. They can also put you in touch with your nearest local contact and provide you with information about their services. The helpline also offers support and information to those supporting bereaved families.

## Cruse Bereavement Care
Cruse House, 126 Sheen Road, Richmond, Surrey TW9 1UR
Tel: 020 8939 9530
National helpline: 08701 671 677
Email: info@crusebereavementcare.org.uk
Website: www.crusebereavementcare.org.uk

Cruse is a charity working to help anyone who has been bereaved. Cruse has 178 branches staffed by 6500 volunteers. Cruse works to increase awareness and understanding of the needs of bereaved people in the community. Cruse provides a range of services including bereavement support, counselling, groups and a national helpline.

## Hospice Information Service
Based at two sites:
Help the Hospices, Hospice House, 34–44 Britannia Street, London WC1X 9JG
and
St Christopher's Hospice, 51–59 Lawrie Park Road, London SE26 6DZ
Tel: 08709 033 903 (calls charged at national rates)
Fax: 020 7278 1021
Email: info@hospiceinformation.info
Website: www.hospiceinformation.info

The Hospice Information Service provides an enquiry service, directories of UK and international hospice and palliative care services, electronic news bulletins, a quarterly magazine and listings of educational and job opportunities.

**Institute for Complementary Medicine**
PO Box 194, London SE16 7QZ
Tel: 020 7237 5165
Email: info@i-c-m.org.uk
Website: www.i-c-m.org.uk

The Institute for Complementary Medicine (ICM) aims to offer the public safe complementary medicine. The ICM established an interdisciplinary register – the British Register of Complementary Practitioners. Only practitioners who have proved to the Registration Panel that they are competent to practise can register. In addition, the ICM affiliates and accredits courses in complementary medicine, has a website containing useful contacts, and a free online journal.

**Institute of Family Therapy**
24–32 Stephenson Way, London NW1 2HX
Tel: 020 7391 9150
Email: ift@psyc.bbk.ac.uk
Website: www.instituteoffamilytherapy.org.uk

The Institute of Family Therapy (IFT) specialises in working with families, individuals, couples and other relationship groups. The service is available to clients who wish to work on their relationships. The IFT have a Family Mediation Service.

**Institute of Psychosexual Medicine**
12 Chandos Street, Cavendish Square, London W1G 9DR
Tel/Fax: 020 7580 0631
Email: admin@ipm.org.uk ; referral: referrals@ipm.org
Website: www.ipm.org.uk

The Institute of Psychosexual Medicine (IPM) is a training organisation for doctors. Seminar training is provided for medical practitioners who come into contact with patients who present with sexual problems. The IPM can provide a list of accredited doctors who accept psychosexual referrals. Please email *referral* or send a stamped addressed envelope stating the area in which you live.

**Let's Face It**
72 Victoria Avenue, Westgate-on-Sea, Kent CT8 8BH
Tel: 01843 833724
Fax: 01843 835695
Email: chrisletsfaceit@aol.com
Website: www.lets-face-it.org.uk

Let's Face It is an international support network linking people with facial disfigurement, their families, friends and professionals with resources for recovery. It aims to:

- offer the hand of friendship on a one-to-one basis
- link families, friends and professionals
- assist people with facial disfigurement to share their experiences, struggles and hopes
- help them build the courage to face life again

- provide continuing education to medical, nursing and allied health professionals concerning the lifelong needs of people with facial disfigurement
- educate the public to value the person behind the face.

**Macmillan Cancer Support**
89 Albert Embankment, London SE1 7UQ
Switchboard: 020 7840 7840
CancerLine: 08088 082 020
Benefits Helpline: 08088 010 301
Email: cancerline@macmillan.org.uk
Website: www.macmillan.org.uk

Macmillan Cancer Support provides information, emotional support, financial assistance and other practical services to people affected by cancer, including specialist health professionals such as Macmillan nurses and doctors. Macmillan has created more than 100 care and treatment centres in hospitals and the community. Macmillan is also working with patients, carers, health and social care professionals, the NHS and the government to shape the future of cancer care.

**Marie Curie Cancer Care**
89 Albert Embankment, London SE1 7TP
Tel: 020 7599 7777
Email: info@mariecurie.org.uk
Website: www.mariecurie.org.uk

Cancer is the UK's biggest killer, claiming the lives of more than 150 000 people annually. Marie Curie Cancer Care is challenging the disease through cancer care and research. Every year the charity provides care to around 25 000 cancer patients and their families at home and in its hospices – entirely free of charge.

**Motor Neurone Disease Association**
PO Box 246, Northampton NN1 2PR
Tel: 01604 250 505
Care information: 01604 611 870
Helpline: 08457 626 262
Email: helpline@mndassociation.org
Website: www.mndassociation.org

The Motor Neurone Disease Association aims to support people living with motor neurone disease to make informed choices and to achieve a quality of life. Their services include equipment loan/financial support, a local branch network, regional support workers as well as a national helpline.

**Multiple Sclerosis Society**
MS National Centre, 372 Edgware Road, London NW2 6ND
Tel: 020 8438 0700
Helpline: 08088 008 000
Research and Services, general enquiries: 020 8438 0742
PA to Director of Research and Services: 020 8438 0765
Email: info@mssociety.org.uk
Website: www.mssociety.org.uk

The Multiple Sclerosis Society is dedicated to a vision of a world without multiple sclerosis (MS), funding and promoting the highest quality research into MS. They also support everyone affected by MS by providing a range of services including welfare grants, information, education and training, MS nurses and a freephone helpline.

**National Association of Bereavement Services**
20 Norton Folgate, London E1 6DB
Tel: 020 7247 0617
Referral helpline: 020 7247 1080
Fax: 020 7247 0617
Website: www.thegrovesurgery.co.uk/shbereav.html

The National Association of Bereavement Services is a coordinating body for bereavement and loss services and acts as a referral agency by enabling bereaved and grieving people to be in touch with their nearest and most appropriate local service. The association's aims and objectives include:

- to compile a national directory of bereavement services
- to initiate and encourage regional support groups for those involved in Bereavement Services
- to provide a forum for members of the association
- to arrange training activities for volunteers, counsellors, coordinators and other professional workers
- to undertake and facilitate debate and research on matters related to terminal illness, loss and bereavement and to disseminate the results
- to highlight gaps in provision and to press for new services to be established
- to offer advice and information and to promote awareness of matters relating to the terminally ill and their families and to bereavement.

**National Institute for Health and Clinical Excellence (NICE)**
MidCity Place, 71 High Holborn, London WC1V 6NA
Tel: 020 7067 5800
Fax: 020 7067 5801
Email: nice@nice.org.uk
Website: www.nice.org.uk

NICE is the independent organisation responsible for providing national guidance on the promotion of good health and the prevention and treatment of ill health.

**Outsiders Trust**
Dr Tuppy Owens
BCM Box Lovely, London WC1N 3XX
Tel: 07074 993527
Email: outsiders@clara.co.uk

and

**Outsiders**
BCM Box Outsiders, London WC1N 3XX
Tel: 020 7354 8291
Email: info@outsiders.org.uk
Website: www.outsiders.org.uk

and

**Sex and Disability Helpline**
Dr Tuppy Owens
BCM Box Lovely, London WC1N 3XX
Tel: 07074 993527
Email: SexAndDisabilityHelpline@gmail.com
Website: www.outsiders.org.uk

Outsiders is a nationwide, self-help community providing regular mailings and unthreatening events where people meet up and practise socialising. Members appreciate a club where they are totally accepted, and some of the most amazing relationships have been formed. Outsiders is for people who feel isolated because of social and physical disabilities. The club helps them gain confidence, make new friends and find partners. Outsiders welcomes people of all sexualities, whether they are single, divorced, separated or married, and discriminates against no one. Members appreciate a club where disability is accepted and people can relax and be themselves. The first step may be to acknowledge the person's sexuality, and offer support in asserting their right to a private life, and seeking love in a society where status normally stems from good looks and money.

**Parkinson's Disease Society of the UK**
215 Vauxhall Bridge Road, London SW1V 1EJ
Tel: 020 7931 8080
Fax: 020 7233 9908
Helpline: 08088 000 303 (9:30 am to 5:30 pm, Monday to Friday)
Email: enquiries@parkinsons.org.uk
Website: www.parkinsons.org.uk

The Parkinson's Disease Society is dedicated to supporting all people with Parkinson's, their families, friends and carers. For advice, information or support, call the helpline.

**Relate**
Herbert Gray College, Little Church Street, Rugby CV21 3AP
Tel: 08454 561 310
RelateLine: 08451 304 010 (helpline where you can get to talk for 20 minutes with a Relate counsellor, open 9:30 am to 4:30 pm, Monday to Friday)
Relate Direct: 08451 304 016 (telephone counselling service)
Email: Enquiries@relate.org.uk
Website: www.relate.org.uk

Relate is the leading national provider of relationship support for couples and families. Relate works with individual families, agencies and employers to help people manage relationship issues.

**Sacred Space Foundation**
Contact: Jean Sayre-Adams
Emmers Farm, Sparket, Penrith, Cumbria CA11 0NA
Tel: 017684 86868
Email: Jeannie@sacredspace.org.uk
Website: www.sacredspace.org.uk

The Sacred Space Foundation provides retreat facilities and psycho/spiritual counselling (if desired) for those who are stressed, burnt out and searching for meaning in their lives. They have two sites in the Lake District. The focus is on healthcare professionals, but they accept others if space allows.

**Stroke Association**
240 City Road, London EC1V 2PR
Tel: 020 7566 0300
Helpline: 08453 033 100 (9 am to 5 pm, Monday to Friday)
Email: info@stroke.org.uk
Website: www.stroke.org.uk

The Stroke Association is a charity for people of all ages affected by stroke. They provide information and support through their helpline and community support services, fund research into all aspects of stroke and campaign to raise awareness of stroke and to improve stroke services.

**Terence Higgins Trust/Lighthouse**
52–54 Grays Inn Road, London WC1X 8JU
Tel: 020 7831 0330
Helpline THT Direct: 08451 221 200 (10 am to 10 pm, Monday to Friday; 12 pm to 6 pm, Saturday to Sunday)
Fax: 020 7242 0121
Email: info@tht.org.uk
Website: www.tht.org.uk

The Terence Higgins Trust is the HIV (human immunodeficiency virus) and sexual health charity, providing a wide range of services to over 50 000 people a year. The charity campaigns and lobbies for greater political and public understanding of the personal, social and medical impact of HIV and sexual health.

# Index

Page numbers in *italic* refer to figures or tables.